D0175096

# *Mayo Clinic on*
# *Prostate Health*

**Michael Blute, M.D.**

Editor in Chief

Mayo Clinic

Rochester, Minnesota

*Mayo Clinic on Prostate Health* provides reliable, practical, easy-to-understand information on identifying and managing prostate conditions. Much of this information comes directly from the experience of doctors, nurses, research scientists, therapists and other health care professionals at Mayo Clinic. This book supplements the advice of your physician, whom you should consult for individual medical problems. *Mayo Clinic on Prostate Health* does not endorse any company or product. MAYO, MAYO CLINIC, MAYO CLINIC HEALTH INFORMATION and the Mayo triple-shield logo are registered marks of Mayo Foundation for Medical Education and Research.

Published by Mayo Clinic Health Information, Rochester, Minn. Distributed to the book trade by Kensington Publishing Corporation, New York, N.Y.

Photo credits: Cover photos and the photos on pages 1, 25, 61 and 141 are from PhotoDisc.

Library of Congress Catalog Card Number: 2003107390

ISBN 1-893005-28-3

Printed in the United States of America

Second Edition

2 3 4 5 6 7 8 9 10

## About prostate disease

Odds are that if you're a man, sooner or later you'll experience a prostate problem. Prostate disease affects more than half of all men and becomes more prevalent with age. Inflammation, enlargement and cancer of the prostate gland are three typical problems men face. Although annoying and sometimes painful, inflammation and enlargement generally aren't life-threatening. Prostate cancer, on the other hand, is now the most common form of life-threatening cancer in men. However, with early diagnosis, it can often be successfully treated and cured.

Within these pages you'll find practical information you can use to recognize and treat prostate problems before they become difficult to manage or a threat to your life. You'll also learn about lifestyle changes that may reduce your risk of prostate disease. This book is based on the expertise of Mayo Clinic doctors and the advice they give every day while caring for their patients.

## About Mayo Clinic

Mayo Clinic evolved from the frontier practice of Dr. William Worrall Mayo, and the partnership of his two sons, William J. and Charles H. Mayo, in the early 1900s. Pressed by the demands of their busy practice in Rochester, Minn., the Mayo brothers invited other physicians to join them, pioneering the private group practice of medicine. Today, with more than 2,000 physicians and scientists at its three major locations in Rochester, Minn., Jacksonville, Fla., and Scottsdale, Ariz., Mayo Clinic is dedicated to providing comprehensive diagnoses, accurate answers and effective treatments.

With its depth of knowledge, experience and expertise, Mayo Clinic occupies an unparalleled position as a health information resource. Since 1983, Mayo Clinic has published reliable health information for millions of consumers through award-winning newsletters, books and online services. Revenue from the publishing activities supports Mayo Clinic programs, including medical education and research.

## Editorial staff

**Editor in Chief**
Michael Blute, M.D.

**Managing Editor**
Richard Dietman

**Proofreading**
Miranda Attlesey
Donna Hanson

**Editorial Research**
Anthony Cook
Danielle Gerberi
Deirdre Herman
Michelle Hewlett

**Contributing Writers**
Rebecca Gonzalez-Campoy
Lynn Madsen
D.R. Martin
Stephen Miller

Catherine Stroebel
Doug Toft
Susan Wichmann

**Creative Director**
Daniel Brevick

**Design**
Craig King

**Illustration**
Brian Fyffe
Stephen Graepel
John Hagen
M. Alice McKinney
James Postier

**Indexing**
Larry Harrison

## Contributing editors and reviewers

Brent Bauer, M.D.
Patrick Burch, M.D.
Brian Davis, M.D.
Christopher Frye
Donald Hensrud, M.D.
Bradley Leibovich, M.D.

Michael Lieber, M.D.
Lance Mynderse, M.D.
Jennifer K. Nelson, R.D.
David Swanson
John Ward, M.D.

# Preface

Since the first edition of *Mayo Clinic on Prostate Health* was published three years ago, progress has continued in the diagnosis and treatment of prostate disease. Refined minimally invasive techniques and advances in medications have helped make prostate enlargement a more tolerable condition. And advances in surgical techniques, radiation therapy and hormone therapy have contributed to greater success in treating and curing prostate cancer.

But despite advances, prostate disease continues to affect many men as they get older. For example, more than half of men in their 60s and as many as 90 percent of men in their 80s have some signs and symptoms of prostate enlargement. And each year about 220,000 men in the United States are diagnosed with prostate cancer. It remains the second-leading cause of cancer death in men. Prostate cancer, as well as other forms of prostate disease, is often easily treated. The key to a good outcome is early diagnosis. That's why it's so important to know the warning signs of prostate disease and, if you're 50 years or older, that you have a yearly checkup.

In this book, you'll find information on what to expect during a typical prostate checkup. The three common prostate disorders, symptoms that ordinarily accompany each, and various treatment options are all examined in detail. Factors to consider and questions to ask your doctor are included to help you decide the best treatment. The prostate-specific antigen (PSA) screening test also is discussed. An entire chapter is devoted to potential side effects of prostate cancer treatment and how to manage those problems. You'll find ways you may reduce your risk of prostate disease, and the latest on complementary and alternative therapies is also included.

The more you know about prostate disease, the greater are your chances of identifying problems early and making good decisions about treatment. Along with advice from your doctor, this book can help you live a longer, healthier life.

*Michael Blute, M.D.*
Editor in Chief

# Contents

## Part 4: Prostate health

# Part 1

*Prostate basics*

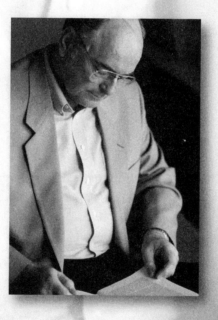

## Chapter 1

# About the prostate

Prostate disease is one of the most common health problems men face, and prostate cancer is among the most feared. That's because prostate cancer, like breast cancer, often affects the core of human sexuality. Beyond the fear of cancer itself are the possible consequences of treatment — bladder control problems (incontinence) and an inability to have an erection (impotence). These conditions can be as difficult as the cancer, shaking confidence and evoking feelings of lost masculinity.

But there's reason for optimism. If caught early, prostate cancer often can be successfully treated and cured. Improved medical practices are reducing the risks of impotence and incontinence. When these conditions do occur, various treatments may limit their effects.

It's also important to understand that cancer isn't the source of all prostate problems. Inflammation and benign enlargement of the prostate are common conditions. Unlike cancer, these problems generally aren't life-threatening, but without early and proper treatment, they can become irritating, debilitating and painful.

For many men as they get older, prostate problems become a fact of life. However, by getting regular checkups and working with your doctor, you can reduce your risk of serious disease and keep your condition from seriously interfering with your routine. This book can help you better understand why prostate problems occur, identify symptoms early, and make informed decisions about treatment.

## A healthy prostate

Found only in men, the prostate gland surrounds the bottom portion (neck) of the bladder. It's located behind the pubic bone and in front of the rectum. About the size and shape of a walnut, the prostate is made up of smooth muscle, spongy tissue, and tiny ducts and glands. Most of its surface is covered by a thin membrane called the capsule.

At birth, the prostate is about the size of a pea. It continues to grow until about age 20, when it reaches adult size. It remains that size until about age 45, when it often begins to grow again.

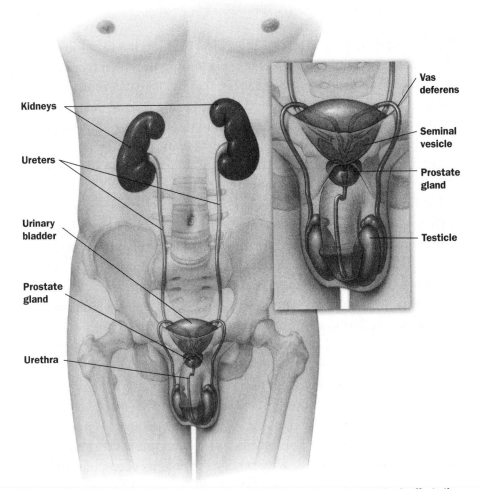

The prostate gland is located deep within the pelvis, just below the urinary bladder. It affects the health of both the reproductive and the urinary systems.

## Reproductive system

The prostate's primary function is to produce most of the fluids in semen, the fluid that transports sperm. Tiny ducts within your prostate carry this fluid to the urethra, the tube that drains fluid from the bladder and out through the penis.

During orgasm, prostate fluid mixes with fluid from the seminal vesicles, located on each side of the prostate, and with sperm to form semen. Sperm travel up from your testicles through long tubes called the vasa deferentia (VA-sa def-uh-REN-shee-uh). Muscle contractions cause ejaculation, during which semen is propelled through the urethra and out of the penis.

To make sure semen doesn't move in the wrong direction and back up into the bladder, a ring of involuntary muscle at the neck of the bladder (internal sphincter) remains tightened during ejaculation. The sphincter also keeps urine from discharging with the semen.

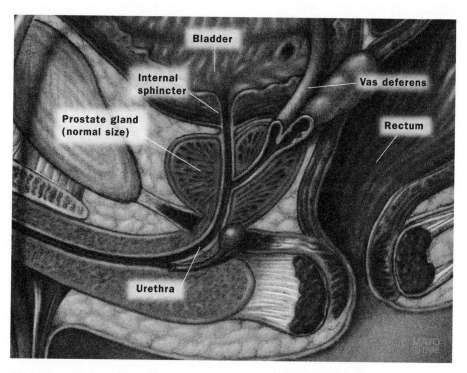

**This cross-sectional view shows the prostate gland and surrounding structures.**

### Urinary system

The prostate gland isn't a primary component of the urinary system, but because of its location, it's important to urinary health.

Your urinary system begins with your kidneys, which cleanse body fluids and produce urine. Urine travels from your kidneys to your bladder through long muscular tubes called ureters (u-REE-turs). Your bladder stores the urine until you urinate. During urination, your bladder muscle contracts and urine exits through the urethra.

Your prostate gland surrounds the top portion of the urethra. Think of your prostate as a small apple with its core missing. The urethra runs through the missing core. When your prostate is healthy, this doesn't pose any problems. But if disease develops in the prostate, tissue in this gland can swell or grow, squeezing the urethra and affecting your ability to urinate.

## When things go wrong

You aren't destined to develop prostate disease. Some men go through life without any prostate problems. Many, however, aren't so lucky. By the time they reach their senior years, a large number of men experience some type of prostate problem. Symptoms may range from minor and mildly annoying to serious and painful.

Three types of diseases can affect the prostate gland. Often, but not always, they occur at different periods in a man's life.

### Inflammation

With this condition, your prostate swells and becomes tender. Many times, a bacterial infection is the source of the inflammation. Other times, the cause is unknown. Called prostatitis (pros-tuh-TIE-tis), prostate inflammation is the most common prostate problem among men under age 50.

### Noncancerous enlargement

Around age 45, tissue inside the prostate gland often begins to grow again. This growth is called benign prostatic hyperplasia (pros-TAT-ik hi-pur-PLA-zhuh), or BPH. It typically occurs in the center portion of the gland, causing prostate tissue to press on the urethra and produce urinary problems. It's the most common prostate problem for men age 50 and older.

### Cancer

Prostate cancer most often occurs after age 50. Prostate cancer results from abnormal and uncontrolled growth of tissue cells. Unlike BPH, in which most of the growth is in the innermost region of the gland, with prostate cancer, tumors generally develop in the outer portion of the prostate. Depending on the type of cancer, these tumors may grow very slowly or at a more rapid pace.

## Symptoms that may signal a problem

Irritating or painful symptoms will often alert you to a prostate problem. This is especially true of prostate inflammation or enlargement.

The following signs and symptoms are often associated with prostate disease. However, they aren't limited to the prostate. Other conditions, such as a urinary infection, bladder problems or kidney stones, can produce some of the same signs and symptoms:

- Excessive urination at night (nocturia)
- Difficulty starting your urine stream
- Decreased strength and force of your urine stream
- Urinating more frequently
- Feeling as if your bladder isn't empty, even after you've just urinated
- Interrupted flow of urine stream
- Dribbling after you've finished urinating
- Urgent need to urinate
- Blood in your urine (hematuria)
- Painful ejaculation
- Pain or a burning sensation while urinating
- Tenderness or pain in the pelvis
- Persistent back or hip pain
- Pain or swelling in the testicles

Unfortunately, prostate cancer produces few, if any, symptoms in its early stages. It's not until later, when the disease is more difficult to treat, that symptoms such as urination difficulties or back pain may develop. That's why it's important to have regular prostate checkups to identify the disease early.

## Are you at risk?

There's no simple formula to tell precisely who will encounter prostate problems. However, various factors — some of them controllable, some not — can affect your odds.

### Uncontrollable risk factors

These are the most common risk factors for prostate disease:

**Age.** As you get older, your risk of BPH and prostate cancer increases. It's estimated that more than half the men in the United States between the ages of 60 and 70 and as many as 90 percent between the ages of 70 and 90 have signs and symptoms of BPH. Indeed, it has been said that all men will have BPH if they live long enough.

Prostate cancer also increases in frequency as men get older. More than 70 percent of men diagnosed with prostate cancer are age 65 or older.

**Ethnic group.** For reasons that aren't well understood, black men are more likely to have prostate cancer than are men of any other group. They're also more likely to have prostate cancer at a younger age, and to have an aggressive form. Black men have prostate cancer mortality rates about twice as high as white and Hispanic men, three times as high as Asian-Americans and five times as high as American Indian men. Asian-American men, on the other hand, have the lowest rate of prostate cancer. The rate of prostate cancer in Hispanic and American Indian men is lower than in whites.

**Family history.** Studies show that if your father or brother has prostate cancer, your risk of the disease is at least twice as great as that of the average American male. And depending on the number of relatives with prostate cancer and the age at which they had it, your risk could be even higher. In families with a history of prostate cancer, the cancer generally occurs at a younger age.

Family history may also play a role in risk of BPH. Age is the primary risk factor for the condition. But among men who have BPH in their 40s or early 50s, many carry an inherited gene that predisposes them to the disease. Carrying the gene doesn't mean that disease is inevitable. It simply increases the risk.

**Bone mass.** How much bone mass you have also may influence your risk of prostate cancer. Researchers at the Boston University School of Medicine found that in a group of about 1,000 men followed for about 30 years, those with the highest bone mass were more likely to develop prostate cancer than were men with the lowest amount of bone mass. The scientists concluded that bone mass may be one way to predict the likelihood of developing prostate cancer. The reasons behind the association weren't clear.

### Controllable risk factors

Risk of prostate cancer differs among populations. Because these differences don't appear to be genetic, researchers suspect that environment and lifestyle factors may play a role in your risk of prostate disease. However, at this point, there are more questions regarding what these factors might be than there are answers.

**Environment.** Researchers are studying whether occupational exposure to certain substances may play an important role. Higher death rates from prostate cancer can be found in certain blue-collar workers, such as farmers, mechanics, welders and industrial employees, than can be found in men in other occupations.

A 1999 Mayo Clinic study of more than 1,000 Iowa farmers found that those age 70 and older were about twice as likely to have prostate cancer as were nonfarmers the same age. The study also suggested that the increase may have been due to occupational exposure and not to dietary or lifestyle factors.

**Diet.** There's some evidence that a diet high in fat — particularly in saturated fat — may increase your risk of prostate cancer. Researchers at the Harvard Medical School and the Harvard School of Public Health evaluated the diets of more than 50,000 health professionals for four years. They found that the men with high-fat diets were nearly twice as likely to have prostate cancer as were men who ate less fat.

Diets high in total calories also may increase risk of prostate cancer. Researchers at the Fred Hutchinson Cancer Research Center in Seattle surveyed dietary habits of nearly 1,200 participants during a three-to-five year period. In a study published in 2002, they concluded that men with a high intake of calories had an increased risk of prostate cancer, as did men with diets high in fat and calcium. A study published in 2003 by researchers at Johns Hopkins Bloomberg School of Public Health also found a link between a high total calorie intake and prostate cancer risk.

Researchers theorize that the increased risk may be because fat increases production of the hormone testosterone, which in turn speeds development of prostate cancer cells. If this theory proves correct, you may be able to reduce your risk of prostate cancer, or slow its development, by limiting fat in your diet. The Seattle researchers concluded that men can reduce their risk of prostate cancer by 50 percent by limiting fat intake to less than 30 percent of their daily caloric intake.

There's also evidence that chemicals found in soy products and certain vegetables and fruits may lower your risk of prostate cancer. See Chapter 11 for different ways — including diet — in which you may be able to protect yourself against prostate disease or delay its development.

**Sexual activity.** Men with a history of sexually transmitted diseases (STDs) may be at higher risk of prostate cancer. In a study published in the journal *Epidemiology,* researchers analyzed 36 studies that evaluated the possible link between STDs and prostate cancer. They found that men with a history of any STD were between 1.4 and 2.3 times as likely to develop prostate cancer as were men without such histories.

The number of sex partners men have during their teens, 20s, 40s and between the ages of 50 and 64 may also increase their risk of prostate cancer. Researchers at the University of Illinois concluded that having two or more female partners during these periods increased the risk of cancer. They also found that men who had 30

# YOU DOCS: Avoid red meat, sugars to lower PSA

FROM PAGE D1

to 30 percent of high PSAs actually mean prostate cancer. First, get a retest. An infection or even a roll in the hay shortly beforehand could have temporarily boosted your PSA level. Also, ask about "percent free" PSA, a type that floats around in your blood, unattached to other molecules. The less you have, the lower your cancer risk.

**5.** What if you get a scary diagnosis? Don't rush to radical surgery. Get a second and maybe third opinion. Up to 40 percent of guys with early prostate cancer can opt for "active surveillance," which monitors the cancer with regular PSAs, prostate exams and biopsies. If trouble arises, treatment starts. We love this approach because it lets you make healthy changes that are proven to keep PSA levels lower even after a cancer diagnosis. The changes: more fruit and veggies, more workouts, more meditation; no red meat, no added sugars and no syrups. Follow these — especially the "no's" — as if your life depended on them. It may.

## NICE TO KNOW

According to the Commission for Certification in Geriatric Pharmacy, patients age 65 and older account for 48 percent of all in-patient hospital stays.

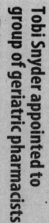

### Tobi Snyder appointed to group of geriatric pharmacists

Tobi Snyder of Windsor, a clinical pharmacist at McKee Medical Center, has been appointed to the Board of Commissioners for The Commission for Certification in Geriatric Pharmacy.

The international organization certifies knowledgeable and committed pharmacists who specialize in the pharmaceutical care of the elderly.

There are only about 1,700 certified ge

or more sexual partners in their lifetime had an increased risk of more aggressive prostate cancer.

**Tobacco.** Cigarette smoking may increase the risk of prostate cancer in younger men. In a study published in 2003 in *The Journal of Urology*, researchers found that among men younger than 55 who'd had their prostate glands removed because of cancer, current smokers were three times as likely as were nonsmokers to have an advanced form of the disease. The researchers also found that the longer the men had smoked before being diagnosed, the more likely they were to have higher-risk prostate cancer. Higher-risk disease was defined as cancer that had spread beyond the prostate.

**Supplemental hormones.** Large doses of the nutritional supplement dehydroepiandrosterone (DHEA) may aggravate prostate enlargement or promote development of prostate cancer. DHEA is a hormone that occurs naturally in your body. It's thought to be a precursor hormone that's easily converted into other hormones, such as testosterone and estrogen. DHEA levels in your body increase sharply at puberty, peak during adulthood and then decrease gradually as you age.

DHEA supplements are promoted to slow aging, burn fat, build muscle and strengthen the immune system. They're also touted as a treatment for various illnesses, including Alzheimer's disease and Parkinson's disease. Studies so far haven't proved that the supplements provide benefits. Their long-term effects and how they may interact with other drugs also are uncertain.

## Answers to your questions

*Is it possible to be born with an abnormal prostate gland?*
Yes. You can have a congenital abnormality in your prostate. Because of the location where the prostate develops, men with congenital prostate abnormalities sometimes also have kidney abnormalities. These conditions aren't common, however, and they can easily be ruled out through X-ray or ultrasound images of the prostate gland and the kidneys.

*I once had a sexually transmitted disease. Does this increase my risk of
prostate problems?*
Possibly. Some sexually transmitted diseases, such as gonorrhea
and chlamydia, may cause inflammation in your urethra, the tube
that carries urine out of your bladder. This inflammation can sometimes produce scar tissue that can narrow or block the urethra,
increasing your risk of urinary infections or infection in your
prostate gland (prostatitis).

*Is it true that a vasectomy can increase my risk of prostate cancer?*
No. A few studies raised speculation that having a vasectomy may
increase the risk of prostate cancer. However, researchers with
the National Institutes of Health have reviewed data on vasectomies and concluded that the sterilization procedure doesn't
increase a man's risk of getting prostate cancer.

Researchers believe that the questions raised in the studies can
be explained by the fact that most vasectomies are done by
urologists, and that men who have a good relationship with a
urologist are more likely to get regular prostate checkups.
Therefore, their cancer is detected earlier than that of men who
don't get regular prostate examinations.

## Chapter 2

# Getting a prostate checkup

You are your own best protection against prostate disease. If you can help identify the condition in its early stages, you have a good chance of successful treatment. How do you do that? With regular prostate checkups.

No specific schedule exists for when to begin having prostate checkups. If you're in your 20s or 30s, a yearly exam generally isn't necessary, unless you have a family history of prostate disease or you're experiencing prostate-related symptoms.

Once you reach your 50s, however, you'll want to consider having a prostate examination yearly and continue to have regular checkups throughout your lifetime. What's involved in a typical exam will vary, depending on your age, doctor, family history and test results.

## Basic diagnostic tests

Most men have a prostate checkup in conjunction with their regular physical examination. In addition to standard procedures and tests that go along with a physical exam, such as checking your blood pressure and listening to your lungs, you may have some or all of the following:

### Digital rectal examination

The digital rectal examination (DRE) is a basic and easy screening test for prostate disease. However, it may rank among the least-desirable parts of a physical exam for many men because it seems embarrassing or they find it uncomfortable.

To perform the exam, your doctor puts on an examination glove and applies a lubricant to one finger. You're then asked to bend forward — perhaps leaning on an examination table — and your doctor gently inserts the lubricated finger into your rectum.

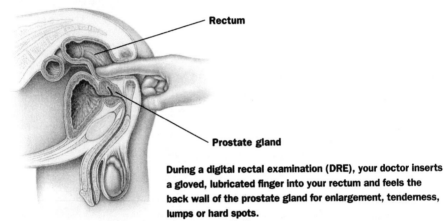

**Rectum**

**Prostate gland**

During a digital rectal examination (DRE), your doctor inserts a gloved, lubricated finger into your rectum and feels the back wall of the prostate gland for enlargement, tenderness, lumps or hard spots.

Because the prostate gland is located adjacent to the rectum, your doctor can feel the back wall of the gland with his or her finger. A gland that feels enlarged may indicate benign prostatic hyperplasia (BPH). If the gland feels tender to the touch, it may be a sign of prostatitis. In addition, the outer portion of the gland is where 70 percent to 85 percent of cancerous tumors develop. In their early stages, they often feel like nodules or hard spots. If your doctor detects such an abnormality, it doesn't necessarily mean you have cancer, but he or she may want to perform additional tests. Other conditions, including a prostate infection or formation of small stones in the gland, can produce similar characteristics.

A Mayo Clinic study published in 1998 found strong evidence that men who didn't receive regular DREs were more likely to die of prostate cancer than were a similar group of men who did have regular exams. The researchers believe that timely DREs could have saved the lives of 50 percent to 70 percent of these men.

Opinions differ among health care organizations as to when men should begin having DREs. Some groups recommend age 50, others age 40. Mayo Clinic urologists agree with the recommendation of the American Urological Association (AUA) that unless a man is at high risk, he should have a yearly DRE beginning at age 50.

## Urine test

This test looks for abnormalities in your urine that may indicate a problem. If your urine contains more white blood cells than is normal, you may have an infection in your prostate gland or urinary tract.

Red blood cells in your urine may signal inflammation of the prostate or, perhaps, a tumor. Other conditions, including bladder problems or inflammation of the urethra, also can produce blood in your urine. In addition, if your doctor thinks you have BPH, a urine test result that's normal can help confirm the diagnosis.

## Blood test

A small amount of blood is drawn from your arm and analyzed for a substance called prostate-specific antigen (PSA). The antigen is produced in your prostate gland to help liquefy semen. A small amount of it, however, enters your bloodstream and circulates in your blood. If higher-than-normal levels of PSA are detected in your blood, it could indicate prostate inflammation, enlargement or cancer.

Most men first have a PSA test between the ages of 40 and 50. In the next sections of this chapter, the PSA test and the controversy surrounding it are discussed in detail.

## Ultrasound

If your doctor has some concerns about the results of your digital rectal exam or urine or blood tests, he or she may want to take a closer look at your prostate gland. This can be done with a procedure called a transrectal ultrasound.

Ultrasonography is an imaging technique that uses sound waves to see inside your body. It's similar to sonar, except that it uses high-frequency sound waves that are reflected or absorbed to varying degrees, depending on the consistency of an object. Because cancerous tissue is thicker and more dense than healthy tissue, the sound-wave reflections may be different.

During a transrectal ultrasound, your doctor inserts a small, lubricated probe, which emits sound waves, into your rectum. The reflections from the waves are translated by a computer and converted into a video picture. The procedure is harmless, although some men find it a little uncomfortable.

If your doctor doesn't find anything serious, you may not need more tests. If the ultrasound result suggests cancer, a biopsy is needed to confirm its presence.

## More on the prostate-specific antigen test

The prostate-specific antigen (PSA) test was approved by the Food and Drug Administration in 1986 as a means to help detect prostate cancer. Since the test was approved, an increase has been observed in the number of cases of the disease — often in its early stages, when the cancer often can be cured.

After a small amount of blood is taken from your arm, the sample is sent to a laboratory where it's tested with a procedure called an immunochemical assay. This procedure determines how much PSA is circulating in your blood.

A reading between 0 and 4 nanograms per milliliter (ng/mL) is normal. However, because PSA levels tend to increase with a person's age, some medical centers have adjusted their standards based on age (see "Mayo Clinic PSA standards" on the next page).

If your PSA level is above normal, that doesn't necessarily mean you have cancer. Some men have higher-than-normal PSA levels and healthy prostates. Conditions other than cancer can increase the amount of PSA circulating in your blood.

**BPH.** Noncancerous enlargement of the prostate is the most common condition that can lead to an elevated PSA reading. As prostate tissue grows, cells within the tissue produce more PSA — sometimes up to three times higher than normal.

**Prostatitis.** Irritation of the prostate gland due to inflammation or an infection can cause cells to release increased amounts of PSA.

## Mayo Clinic PSA standards

Mayo Clinic urologists use this age-adjusted scale to determine PSA normal upper limits*, based on the test used at Mayo.

| Age | Upper limit ng/mL** | Age | Upper limit ng/mL | Age | Upper limit ng/mL | Age | Upper limit ng/mL |
|---|---|---|---|---|---|---|---|
| ≤ 40 | 2.0 | 51 | 2.9 | 62 | 4.1 | 73 | 5.8 |
| 41 | 2.1 | 52 | 3.0 | 63 | 4.2 | 74 | 6.0 |
| 42 | 2.2 | 53 | 3.1 | 64 | 4.4 | 75 | 6.2 |
| 43 | 2.3 | 54 | 3.2 | 65 | 4.5 | 76 | 6.4 |
| 44 | 2.3 | 55 | 3.3 | 66 | 4.6 | 77 | 6.6 |
| 45 | 2.4 | 56 | 3.4 | 67 | 4.8 | 78 | 6.8 |
| 46 | 2.5 | 57 | 3.5 | 68 | 4.9 | 79 | 7.0 |
| 47 | 2.6 | 58 | 3.6 | 69 | 5.1 | ≥ 80 | 7.2 |
| 48 | 2.6 | 59 | 3.7 | 70 | 5.3 | | |
| 49 | 2.7 | 60 | 3.8 | 71 | 5.4 | | |
| 50 | 2.8 | 61 | 4.0 | 72 | 5.6 | | |

*Upper limits increase almost every year as you age.
**Nanograms per milliliter

**Cancer.** Cancerous cells in the prostate also produce PSA. A higher-than-normal PSA reading may indicate the presence of cancer in prostate tissue.

Other factors also can increase your PSA level. They include:

**Ejaculation.** Ejaculation can cause a temporary increase in the PSA level in your blood. For that reason, some doctors advise their patients to abstain from sexual activity up to two days before having their PSA measured. However, a study published in 1998 found that the increased levels of PSA after ejaculation dropped quickly and weren't considered high enough to result in abnormal test results. The researchers recommended that men not be asked to refrain from sexual activity before having a PSA-screening test.

**Urinary tract infection.** Like an infection in your prostate gland, a urinary tract infection can increase your PSA level.

**Recent prostate treatment.** Procedures used to treat BPH — discussed in Chapter 5 — can temporarily irritate your prostate gland, producing inflammation and above-normal levels of PSA. These procedures include:

- Prostate biopsy
- Transurethral resection of the prostate
- Transurethral incision of the prostate
- Prostate massage
- Microwave therapy of the prostate
- Laser therapy of the prostate

After having one of these procedures, wait from two weeks to two months to have a PSA test. This allows your PSA to return to the level where it was before the procedure.

---

## BPH medications and PSA

Finasteride (Proscar) and dutasteride (Avodart) are medications used to treat benign prostatic hyperplasia (BPH). They shrink the prostate gland by suppressing certain hormones that stimulate prostate growth. Finasteride is the same drug taken to promote hair growth in balding men and is sold under the brand name Propecia.

By altering the level of hormones in the prostate gland, these drugs reduce production of PSA in the gland. The decrease in PSA is about 50 percent after 12 months of treatment and can occur even if you have prostate cancer, which would normally cause a rise in your PSA level.

This raises a question about the accuracy of PSA testing in men who use these medications. Some doctors believe PSA tests aren't beneficial for men taking finasteride or dutasteride. Others, however, believe that the PSA test can still be useful for tracking PSA ranges in men taking these medications, provided the ranges are adjusted. For example, if the normal PSA range for a 70-year-old man is 0 to 5.3 ng/mL, the normal range for a 70-year-old man taking finasteride or dutasteride might be 0 to 2.65 ng/mL.

It's essential for your doctor to be aware if you're taking these medications so that he or she can monitor and interpret the PSA results appropriately.

### How accurate is the PSA test?

The PSA test detects cancer in its early stages about 75 percent of the time. In about 25 percent of men with early prostate cancer, the results come back normal (less than 4 ng/mL). This is one drawback of the test — in about one out of four men with prostate cancer, it may not identify the cancer early if used as the only screening measure.

Another drawback of the PSA test is that it can't distinguish between cancer and other prostate diseases. Among men with an elevated PSA level, only one-third have cancer. Increased PSA levels in the other two-thirds may be the result of BPH, prostatitis or some other factor. As a result, many men who don't have cancer might undergo additional tests to rule out cancer.

## The debate

Not all doctors and medical organizations agree that the benefits of the PSA test outweigh its limitations. That's why this simple test is a controversial screening tool.

### Benefits

Regular PSA screening can help identify prostate cancer long before any signs or symptoms become apparent. The PSA test is often able to detect cancer when it's still confined to the prostate gland. Localized cancer is much easier to treat and cure than cancer that has spread to other organs and tissues.

Not all prostate cancers are alike. Some grow very slowly and remain within the prostate gland. Others are more aggressive and can spread rather quickly to other organs. If your PSA test detects what turns out to be an aggressive form of prostate cancer, it could literally be a lifesaver.

The year 1995 marked the first-ever reduction in deaths from prostate cancer. Many doctors believe, and some studies confirm, that the PSA test was a major factor behind the decrease. However, health experts haven't been able to prove with certainty that the screening test reduces prostate cancer deaths.

## Limitations

The PSA test isn't completely reliable. In about 25 percent of men in whom the test fails to identify prostate cancer, it may give a false sense of security about their prostate health. And among men with an elevated PSA, approximately two out of three may go through needless worry and unnecessary, expensive diagnostic procedures.

Whether the test leads to needless treatment is another question. If you have a slow-growing cancer, you may be able to live with it for years without it causing any problems. For some men, this can be difficult to accept. When they learn they have cancer, they want to do something to get rid of it, such as undergo surgery or radiation therapy. These treatments may produce side effects, including incontinence or impotence. The result can be a decrease in the quality of life for men who might otherwise live healthy, productive lives.

Finally, the issue of whether early detection and treatment of prostate cancer actually saves lives remains to be resolved. A Swedish study published in 2002 found that in a group of men whose average age was 65, surgical treatment of early prostate cancer reduced prostate cancer deaths. However, the same study found that after a six-year follow-up period, the mortality rates for all causes were fairly similar both in the group that received treatment and the group that didn't.

## A final answer?

Two large, long-term studies now under way in the United States may provide some answers and help settle the PSA debate. However, it will be several years before the results are known.

**PLCO.** The Prostate, Lung, Colorectal and Ovarian Cancer Screening Trial is a large study sponsored by the National Cancer Institute to determine whether screening and early detection of cancer save lives. For prostate cancer, men are screened once a year for four years and then followed for 12 more years.

**PIVOT.** The Prostate cancer Intervention Versus Observations Trial was begun in 1994 and is funded by the Department of Veterans Affairs and the National Cancer Institute.

The goal of PIVOT is to determine the best way to treat cancer confined to the prostate gland — whether to perform surgery to remove the gland or let the gland alone and watch to see if the cancer spreads (watchful waiting). Participants in the study have regular examinations and periodically fill out questionnaires regarding their quality of life.

### Current recommendations

So, in the meantime, should you have a PSA test?

There's no definitive answer. Of the medical organizations that have taken a stand on the PSA test, about one-third support its use, one-third are neutral, and one-third don't support it.

The American Cancer Society (ACS), the National Comprehensive Cancer Network and the AUA are among its supporters. The ACS recommends that the PSA test — along with the DRE — be offered annually to all men beginning at age 50. It also recommends that because they are at higher risk, black men begin testing at age 45. And the ACS recommends that men with a family history of prostate cancer begin screening at age 40.

As for how long you continue to take the test, the ACS and AUA recommend lifelong screening. Many men in their 70s remain in excellent health and have good quality of life. They may have a life expectancy of at least 15 years and consequently might benefit from routine PSA testing. Other organizations, however, suggest that after age 70 the test may no longer be necessary, particularly in cases where life expectancy is determined to be less than 10 years.

The American Medical Association (AMA) recommends that men be informed of the potential benefits and shortcomings of prostate cancer screening and that the PSA test should be made available to informed patients who request it. The AMA has declined to endorse mass screening for prostate cancer.

### Mayo Clinic's view

Mayo Clinic prostate cancer specialists understand the pitfalls of the PSA test and agree that it's not perfect. But they support its use — along with the DRE — because it's the best screening tool available for detecting prostate cancer in its early stages. It's especially beneficial for younger men who have more curable cancers. As with many other cancers, the earlier prostate cancer is found, the greater your chance for a complete recovery. Early detection also allows time to make good treatment decisions.

In accordance with the ACS and the AUA, Mayo Clinic specialists recommend an annual PSA test beginning at age 50, unless you're at high risk of prostate cancer. If you're black or you have a family history of prostate cancer, you may want to begin at age 40.

If you have concerns about the PSA test — such as what are your chances of getting a false result, what should you do if you have a high PSA reading, and whether you're too old to have the test — discuss them with your doctor.

## In search of a better screening tool

Researchers continue to look for a more accurate and specific screening test for prostate cancer that can reduce or eliminate some disadvantages of the PSA test. Several options are being studied:

**Free-PSA test.** PSA comes in two forms — PSA that's bound by blood proteins and PSA that's unbound, called free PSA. The current test measures both bound and unbound PSA to determine the total amount of PSA in your blood. Researchers have learned, however, that cancer is more likely to produce bound PSA, whereas BPH is linked to an increase in free PSA.

The free-PSA test indicates how much PSA circulates by itself in the blood and how much is bound together with blood proteins. The lower the percentage of free PSA, the more likely that cancer may be responsible for the increase in your PSA level. The higher the percentage of free PSA, the greater the chance BPH may be the cause (see "Free-PSA test" chart on the next page).

**PSA velocity test.** This test charts the rate of change in your PSA levels. Scientists believe that the number of PSA molecules increases more quickly in someone with prostate cancer than in someone with BPH or prostatitis.

**PSA density test.** Prostate-specific antigen density (PSAD) is determined by dividing your PSA level by your prostate volume. Your prostate volume can be obtained by ultrasound. A higher PSAD generally indicates a greater likelihood of cancer.

**Ultrasensitive PSA test.** This specialized test is capable of detecting minute quantities of PSA in your bloodstream. If you've already been treated for prostate cancer, the test may detect a recurrence of cancer far earlier than is possible with other tests — perhaps by one or two years.

**Other markers.** A number of other substances similar to PSA may serve as markers for early-stage prostate cancer. They include human glandular kallikrein, chromogranin A, and prostate-specific membrane antigen (PSMA). Screening tests for these sub-

## Free-PSA test

The first table shows the probability of detecting cancer by needle biopsy based on your total PSA level.

| Total PSA (ng/mL) | % Probability of cancer |
|:---:|:---:|
| 0 to 2 | about 1 |
| 2 to 4** | 15 |
| 4 to 10 | 25 |

To further determine the probability of cancer when total PSA is in the 4 to 10 ng/mL range, your doctor may evaluate your free-PSA level. The higher the percent of free-PSA, the lower the probability of cancer.*

| % Free PSA | % Probability of cancer |
|:---:|:---:|
| 0 to 10 | 56 |
| 10 to 15 | 28 |
| 15 to 20 | 20 |
| 20 to 25 | 16 |
| over 25 | 8 |

*Data are for men with normal digital rectal examination results, regardless of age.

**Normal PSA values may be less for younger men.

Adapted from *The Journal of the American Medical Association*, May 20, 1998.

stances could eventually prove to be more reliable indicators of prostate cancer than the current PSA test.

A number of new tests that measure the distribution of various proteins in the blood — called serum proteomic patterns — may lead to a more accurate method of determining whether someone with a high PSA level actually has prostate cancer. Such a test might be used instead of a biopsy, to confirm the presence of disease. One test that measures the level of a protein called EZH2 may help predict the likelihood of recurrence of prostate cancer after the prostate is removed.

**Gene research.** If researchers can identify a gene or genes responsible for prostate cancer, men who carry these genes could be monitored more closely to identify cancer in its very early stages. These men may even be able to prevent cancer through lifestyle changes, including a change in diet.

## Answers to your questions

*Can my family physician do a prostate examination?*
Absolutely. Family physicians are vital to the process of screening men for prostate cancer or other abnormalities. The DRE and PSA test are routine and virtually every family doctor is familiar with them.

*When should I see a urologist?*
Your family doctor may recommend that you see a urologist if he or she has questions regarding your test results, suspects prostate cancer, or believes that a urologist could better treat non-cancerous conditions, such as BPH or prostatitis. If you have a problem urinating, your PSA level is elevated, or your family doctor finds an abnormality during a DRE, you may want to see a urologist.

*Can I request a PSA test if my doctor doesn't routinely give me one?*
Yes. Most health plans allow you to obtain the medical tests you desire. However, the plan may not pay for the test. You may want to check with your doctor and your insurance provider to clarify whether a PSA test is covered by your insurance plan before requesting it. A PSA test costs less than $100.

*My PSA level has always been very low. It's still within the normal range, but it has increased. Should I be concerned?*
As you age, your PSA level may increase slightly. However, a noticeable change in your PSA should be followed with a thorough evaluation, even if the reading is normal.

# Part 2

## Noncancerous conditions

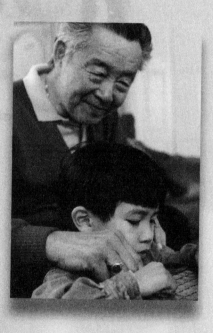

## Chapter 3

# Living with prostatitis

One of the most common prostate problems men encounter is one you seldom hear about — unless you're a doctor. According to some estimates, up to a quarter of all visits men make to a doctor for genital or urinary problems are related to prostatitis. This condition is not only common — it's estimated that as many as 50 percent of men will experience an episode of prostatitis at some point in life — but also can be both tough to diagnose and difficult to treat.

*Prostatitis* is a general term for inflammation of the prostate gland. The inflammation may be due to an infection or another factor that's irritating the gland. Although many things are unclear about the disease, doctors have found that an accurate diagnosis is crucial to treating it. That's because prostatitis can occur in at least three forms.

### Acute bacterial
This is the least common and most severe form of the disease. It results from an infection in the prostate gland that produces severe and often sudden signs and symptoms. These may include a combination of:
- Fever
- Chills
- A general flu-like feeling

- Pain in the lower back and genital area
- Pain or a burning sensation when urinating
- Inability to urinate or decreased urine flow
- Inability to empty the bladder during urination
- A frequent and sometimes urgent need to urinate
- Blood-tinged urine
- Painful ejaculation

Bacteria commonly found in the urinary tract or large intestine are most often responsible for this type of prostatitis. Because acute bacterial prostatitis can lead to serious problems, including an inability to urinate and infection in the bloodstream (bacteremia), it's important that you see a doctor right away. If your symptoms are severe, you may need to be hospitalized for a few days until they improve.

### Chronic bacterial

This condition also is caused by a bacterial infection. However, unlike acute prostatitis, signs and symptoms typically develop more slowly and they're often less severe. They may include:

- Frequent urination
- A sudden or compelling urge to urinate
- Pain or a burning sensation when urinating
- Excessive nighttime urination (nocturia)
- Pain in the lower back and genital area
- Difficulty starting or continuing urination
- A diminished urine flow
- Occasional blood in semen (hematospermia)
- Painful ejaculation
- Slight fever
- Recurring bladder infection

What causes a chronic bacterial infection isn't certain. Like an acute infection, it may result from bacteria in your urinary tract. Other causes may include a bladder or blood infection. The infection may follow trauma to your urinary tract or insertion of an instrument — usually a catheter — into your urethra. That's why some doctors routinely prescribe antibiotics after use of a urinary catheter.

Sometimes, calcified stones can form in your prostate gland and attract bacteria. Rarely, the infection results from an underlying structural defect in your prostate that becomes a collection site for bacteria.

This form of prostatitis is often ongoing (chronic) because the infection can be difficult to get rid of. Antibiotics taken to kill the bacteria have a difficult time penetrating prostate tissues.

### Chronic nonbacterial

Most men with prostatitis have this type. Unfortunately, it's also the most difficult to diagnose and treat. Instead of trying to cure the disease, the main goal of treatment is usually to find relief from the symptoms.

Signs and symptoms of chronic nonbacterial prostatitis are about the same as those for chronic bacterial prostatitis. But one distinguishing factor separates the two: In this kind of prostatitis, your doctor isn't able to detect bacteria in your urine or in fluid from your prostate gland. However, white blood cells in urine specimens signal the presence of inflammation.

The main reason chronic nonbacterial prostatitis is so difficult to diagnose and treat is that its cause is unknown. Theories abound as to possible triggers of the inflammation. However, none is certain and many aren't well understood. Among the possible causes are:

**Sexual activity.** Sexually active younger men with inflammation of the urethra (urethritis) or a sexually transmitted disease, such as gonorrhea or chlamydia, are more likely to develop chronic nonbacterial prostatitis. In some men, a reduction in the frequency of sexual intercourse also may be a contributing factor.

**Other infectious agents.** The inflammation may be related to some kind of infectious agent current tests can't detect.

**Anxiety or stress.** These conditions may cause you to tighten the urinary sphincter muscle, which controls urine flow from the bladder, and those muscles located between your legs that support the bladder and rectum (pelvic floor muscles). Muscle tightening may prevent the muscles from relaxing properly, and may irritate the gland or cause fluids in the urethra to back up into your prostate, irritating inner tissues.

**Heavy lifting.** Lifting heavy objects while your bladder is full also may cause urine to back up and seep into your prostate.

**Certain occupations.** Occupations that subject the prostate to a great deal of vibration, such as truck driving or riding on heavy equipment, may be associated with chronic nonbacterial infection.

**Recreational activities.** Frequent activities such as bicycling or jogging may irritate the prostate gland.

## What kind do you have?

The two most important steps in diagnosing prostatitis are ruling out other conditions that can cause similar symptoms and determining the type of prostatitis you have.

To do this, your doctor will ask you questions about your symptoms: What are they? Do they come and go, or are they persistent? When did they first occur? Can you recall any changes in your routine or lifestyle about the time they began? Your doctor may also ask you about recent medical procedures, previous infections, your sexual habits, your occupation, and whether you have a family history of prostate problems.

A physical examination generally follows. It may include checking your abdomen and pelvic area for unusual tenderness and a digital rectal examination (DRE) of your prostate gland. An inflamed prostate often feels enlarged and tender to the touch.

During the DRE, your doctor may collect fluid from your prostate gland. To do this, he or she will rub rather vigorously against the gland with a gloved finger, forcing fluid out of the gland and into your urethra. From there it passes through your penis. The fluid is collected and examined under a microscope for signs of an infection or inflammation. This procedure is often referred to as prostate massage or prostate stripping.

A urine sample may be collected and tested for bacteria and white blood cells. White blood cells indicate inflammation. Bacteria point to an infection. If your urine tests positive for both — inflammation and infection — you likely have bacterial prostatitis. If the test finds white blood cells but no bacteria, then you probably have the chronic nonbacterial form. If neither bacteria nor white blood cells are found, your symptoms may be related to other disorders. These could include a condition called prostatodynia, discussed later in this chapter.

# Designing a treatment plan

Once your doctor determines the kind of prostatitis you have, the two of you can work together on a plan for treating the condition, and possibly curing it. Since the cause of chronic nonbacterial prostatitis is often unknown, this form of the disease can be difficult to cure. However, with some patience and experimentation, many men find ways to manage the condition and keep it from interfering seriously with their daily lives.

### Medications

One or more of the following drugs may help eliminate or control your symptoms:

**Antibiotics.** Antibiotics are a traditional first line of treatment for all forms of prostatitis. Your doctor will likely start you off on a drug that fights a broad spectrum of bacteria. Once the specific type of bacterium that's causing your infection has been determined — based on your urine and prostatic fluid samples — you may have a different drug prescribed that's more effective at killing the bacteria.

How long you'll need to take an antibiotic will vary depending on how well your infection responds to the drug. If you have acute disease, you may need medication for only a few weeks. Men with acute bacterial prostatitis may need to be hospitalized in order to receive antibiotics intravenously.

Chronic bacterial prostatitis, on the other hand, is often more resistant to antibiotics, making the drugs less effective. It takes longer to cure the infection, and sometimes it can't be cured. In addition, you may have a relapse as soon as the drug is withdrawn. If this happens, you may need to take a low-dose antibiotic daily for an indefinite period to keep the infection under control.

Even though chronic nonbacterial prostatitis isn't caused by an infection, some doctors will prescribe an antibiotic for a few weeks to see if it helps improve symptoms. If the drug doesn't help, your doctor will recommend that you stop taking it. If your symptoms do improve, your doctor may suggest continuing the medication for a few more weeks. Some people with chronic nonbacterial prostatitis find a continuous, low dose of an antibiotic helps to prevent symptoms or reduce their severity. How or why the medication helps is unknown.

**Alpha blockers.** If you're having difficulty urinating, perhaps due to an obstruction in your urinary tract, your doctor may prescribe an alpha blocker. Alpha blockers help relax the prostate and bladder neck, improving urine flow. Because you're able to eliminate more urine, alpha blockers may reduce the number of times you need to go to the bathroom at night.

**Pain relievers.** Over-the-counter pain relievers, such as aspirin, ibuprofen and acetaminophen, can help relieve pain and discomfort. However, discuss with your doctor how much of the drug to take to avoid side effects.

### Physical therapy

Stretching and relaxing the lower pelvic muscles helps to relieve symptoms in some men. A physical therapist can provide guidance on which exercises are beneficial and how to perform them. Heat, in the form of diathermy, may be included in your treatment sessions. This process uses electrical currents to heat tissues in the muscles, making them more limber and easier to relax. After working with a physical therapist, you continue to do the exercises on your own at home.

Your therapist may also try other relaxation techniques, such as biofeedback. Biofeedback uses technology to teach you how to control certain body responses, including relaxing your muscles. During a biofeedback session, a trained therapist attaches electrodes and other sensors to skin on various parts of your body. The electrodes are attached to a monitor that gives you feedback on bodily functions, including muscle tension. Once the electrodes are in place, the therapist uses relaxation techniques to calm you, reducing muscle tension. You then learn how to produce these changes yourself.

Doctors aren't sure why physical therapy works for prostatitis. They speculate that among some men, tight or irritated muscles may be a contributing factor to the condition.

### Sitz baths

Many men find these baths can relieve their pain and relax the pelvic and lower abdominal muscles. From the German word *sitzen*, meaning "to sit," this type of bath simply involves sitting and soaking the lower half of your body in warm water.

---

## Common but unproven practices

Because chronic prostatitis is difficult to understand and treat, over the years men have experimented with various lifestyle changes to control their symptoms. Some more common practices include:

- Drinking plenty of water
- Limiting alcohol, caffeine and highly spiced foods
- Going to the bathroom at regular intervals
- Having frequent sexual intercourse

Although these practices don't cause any harm, no scientific evidence proves they're beneficial. Studies have yet to show that changes in dietary, bathroom or sexual habits can cure prostatitis or relieve your symptoms.

This doesn't mean, however, that if you find such practices helpful you should discontinue them. For reasons that are unclear, some men find that simple things such as avoiding long periods of sitting or certain foods or beverages seem to improve their condition.

For many men with prostatitis, living with the disease often comes down to limiting those things that seem to make the condition worse and doing others that seem to improve it, without knowing why or how the changes help.

It may take months to get relief from chronic prostatitis. The condition can recur for no apparent reason.

---

When your condition is first diagnosed, your doctor may recommend taking sitz baths two or three times a day for 30 minutes each time. For acute bacterial prostatitis, keep the water temperature below 99 F. If you have chronic disease, temperatures up to 115 F are fine.

### Prostate massage

Massaging the prostate can often help to relieve congestion in the gland due to an infection, and to unplug tiny ducts blocked by bacteria. In addition, massage may improve the effectiveness of antibiotics by making it easier for the drugs to penetrate more deeply into infected tissues.

## When it's not prostatitis

Sometimes, men who see a doctor for what appears to be prostatitis don't have prostatitis but another condition called prostatodynia (pros-tuh-toe-DIN-ee-uh). Men with this condition often refer to their symptoms as pain "down there," meaning anywhere in the genital area. The symptoms typically mimic those of chronic non-bacterial prostatitis. As with chronic nonbacterial prostatitis, urine and prostate fluid samples don't indicate evidence of infection or inflammation.

Rather than being a problem with your prostate gland, prostatodynia may instead stem from your pelvic floor muscles. When you're under stress, you may not completely relax those muscles supporting your bladder and urethra, causing difficulties when you urinate. This theory could explain why most men who have prostatodynia tend to have Type A personalities — hard-driven, tense, stressed. Prostatodynia also seems to occur more frequently among marathon runners, bicyclists, triathletes, weightlifters and truck drivers.

Treatment for prostatodynia is similar in many ways to treatment for chronic nonbacterial prostatitis. Physical therapy to help relax your pelvic floor muscles is generally the first step. Your doctor may also recommend stress management courses to help you learn to reduce and better cope with stress.

An alpha blocker medication to relax muscles in your prostate and bladder neck may also be helpful. Some men remain on the drug indefinitely, because their symptoms return when it's withdrawn. You might also try sitz baths to see if they improve your symptoms.

## Answers to your questions

*Does prostatitis increase my risk of cancer?*
There's no evidence that having acute or chronic prostatitis puts you at greater risk of prostate cancer. Prostatitis does, however, increase the level of prostate-specific antigen (PSA) in your blood. If your PSA level is elevated and you have prostatitis, it's advisable to redo the test after you've been treated with antibiotics. If you have chronic prostatitis, ask your doctor about the value of testing your free-PSA level (see "Free-PSA test" on page 23).

*Can I pass on a prostate infection to my partner during intercourse?*
Prostatitis can result from a sexually transmitted disease, but prostatitis itself isn't contagious. Prostatitis can't be passed on through sexual intercourse, so your partner doesn't have to worry about catching an infection.

*Can prostatitis make me infertile?*
It may. The disease can interfere with the development of semen, making it difficult for the fluid to ejaculate properly during intercourse. Because semen carries sperm, this may lower your fertility rate. A few studies indicate poor sperm quality in some men with prostatitis.

*Is surgery ever used to treat the disease?*
Generally, doctors prefer nonsurgical procedures. But if the disease has drastically affected your fertility or antibiotics aren't able to improve your symptoms, your doctor might recommend surgery. A surgeon may try to open blocked ducts in the gland to relieve congestion and help semen flow more freely. Surgery isn't recommended for chronic nonbacterial disease.

*Can the herb saw palmetto help relieve my symptoms?*
Studies show that saw palmetto may be an effective treatment for noncancerous enlargement of the prostate gland (benign prostatic hyperplasia). However, there's no evidence that this popular herb relieves infection or inflammation associated with prostatitis. Saw palmetto is discussed later in this book on page 160.

## Chapter 4

# Understanding benign prostatic hyperplasia (BPH)

A t birth, your prostate gland is about the size of a pea. It grows slightly during childhood and then at puberty undergoes rather rapid growth. By the time you reach age 20, your prostate is fully developed.

Most men, however, experience a second period of prostate growth. When they reach their mid-40s, cells in the central portion of the gland — where the prostate surrounds the urethra — begin to proliferate more rapidly than normal. As tissues in the area enlarge, they often press on the urethra and obstruct urine flow (see illustration). *Benign prostatic hyperplasia* is the medical term for this condition. It's commonly called BPH.

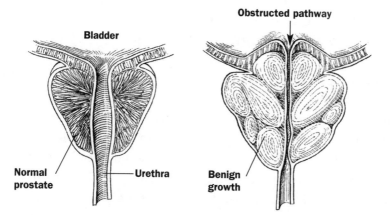

The urethra, the tube that drains the bladder, is surrounded by the prostate gland. Benign prostatic hyperplasia (BPH) results when tissues in the central portion of the prostate gland enlarge and press on the urethra, affecting normal urine flow.

# A fact of life

The chance that you'll develop BPH increases with your age. BPH affects more than half of men in their 60s and about 90 percent of men in their 80s.

The causes of prostate gland enlargement are unclear. Researchers believe that as you age, your prostate becomes more susceptible to the effects of male hormones, including testosterone. These hormones make certain prostate tissues grow.

Other factors likely play a role. A family history of BPH can increase your odds for the disease, pointing to a possible genetic link. BPH is more common in American and European men than in men of Asian descent. This suggests a possible lifestyle component. For unknown reasons, married men are more likely to get BPH than are single men.

The condition varies in severity and doesn't always pose a problem. Only about half the men with BPH experience signs and symptoms that become noticeable or annoying enough for them to seek medical treatment. These signs and symptoms may include:

- Increased urination at night (nocturia)
- A weak urine stream
- Difficulty starting urination
- Stopping and starting again while urinating
- Dribbling at the end of urination
- A frequent or an urgent need to urinate
- Not being able to empty the bladder

Only if it prevents you from emptying your bladder can BPH become a serious health threat. A bladder that's continually full can result in recurrent bladder infection and kidney damage.

BPH doesn't necessarily get worse with time. According to one review, mild to moderate symptoms worsened in only about 20 percent of cases. Symptoms improved in another 20 percent and stayed the same in the remainder of the group.

## Seeing a doctor

If you're experiencing urinary problems, make an appointment to see your doctor, or mention your symptoms at your next visit. Your doctor can determine whether you have BPH and your symptoms require treatment. If you don't find your symptoms annoying and they don't pose a health threat, treatment may not be necessary. That doesn't mean, however, that it's all right to let urinary symptoms go unchecked. Instead of BPH, your symptoms could be early warnings of a more serious condition, including a bladder stone, a bladder infection, bladder cancer, side effects of medication, heart failure, diabetes, a neurologic problem, prostatitis or prostate cancer.

Your doctor will likely begin by asking you questions about your symptoms, when they developed, and how often they occur. He or she will also want to know about other health problems you may have, medications you may be taking, and whether there's a history of prostate problems in your family. In addition, your checkup may include:

- A digital rectal examination to see whether your prostate is enlarged and to help rule out prostate cancer
- A urine test to rule out an infection or a condition that can produce similar symptoms
- A prostate-specific antigen (PSA) test to help rule out prostate cancer.

## Getting a diagnosis

If the results of the previous tests suggest BPH, your doctor may want to perform some additional exams. They can help confirm the diagnosis of BPH and determine its severity.

### American Urological Association Symptom Index

This is a short questionnaire developed by the American Urological Association (AUA). It asks you about specific urinary symptoms associated with BPH and how often they occur (see "How do you rate?" on page 40).

# How do you rate?

The American Urological Association Symptom Index for Benign Prostatic Hyperplasia (BPH) is designed to help doctors evaluate BPH severity.

| Questions | Not at all | Less than 1 time in 5 | Less than half the time | About half the time | More than half the time | Almost always | Score |
|---|---|---|---|---|---|---|---|
| Over the past month, how often have you had a sensation of not emptying your bladder completely after you finished urinating? | 0 | 1 | 2 | 3 | 4 | 5 | ____ |
| Over the past month, how often have you had to urinate again less than two hours after you had finished urinating? | 0 | 1 | 2 | 3 | 4 | 5 | ____ |
| Over the past month, how often have you found you stopped and started again several times when you urinated? | 0 | 1 | 2 | 3 | 4 | 5 | ____ |
| Over the past month, how often have you found it is difficult to postpone urination? | 0 | 1 | 2 | 3 | 4 | 5 | ____ |
| Over the past month, how often have you had a weak urinary stream? | 0 | 1 | 2 | 3 | 4 | 5 | ____ |
| Over the past month, how often have you had to push or strain to begin urination? | 0 | 1 | 2 | 3 | 4 | 5 | ____ |
| | None | 1 time | 2 times | 3 times | 4 times | 5 or more times | |
| Over the past month, how many times did you most typically get up to urinate from the time you went to bed at night until you got up in the morning? | 0 | 1 | 2 | 3 | 4 | 5 | ____ |

**Total Score** ____

## Scoring Key

Mild symptoms: 0 to 7 total points
Moderate symptoms: 8 to 19 total points
Severe symptoms: 20 to 35 total points

Adapted from: American Urological Association Education and Research, 2003

## Bother score

In addition to the AUA's Symptom Index for BPH, the International Prostate Symptoms Score adds a Disease Specific Quality of Life Question to determine how bothered you are by your symptoms. The question asks, "If you were to spend the rest of your life with your urinary condition just the way it is now, how would you feel about that?" The answer, called the bother score, is based on a scale from zero to six, with zero being delighted to six being terrible. You and your doctor may use your bother score to help decide what, if any, treatment is appropriate. For example, someone who has moderate symptoms but a low bother score may be happier with no or minimally invasive treatment rather than with risking potential side effects of a more involved procedure to relieve symptoms. On the other hand, someone with the same symptoms and a high bother score may be willing to tolerate possible side effects of a more invasive treatment in order to get relief.

## Urinary flow test

This test measures the strength and amount of your urine flow. A flow rate of more than 15 milliliters per second (mL/s) is normal or signifies only mild disease. A rate of 10 to 15 mL/s is often associated with moderate symptoms. Anything less than 10 mL/s usually indicates severe BPH. By charting the results of this test, your doctor can determine if your urinary flow patterns are worsening over time, and at what speed. Keep in mind, however, that your flow rate normally decreases as you age. Restricted urine flow can also be a sign of other problems, such as weak bladder muscles.

## Postvoid residual volume test

This test measures whether you can empty your bladder. The test is done one of two ways — by inserting a small catheter into your urethra and up into your bladder or by using ultrasound imaging to see inside your bladder.

## Ultrasound imaging

The ultrasound method of measuring postvoid volume is a more common but less accurate reading. Because the results of this test can vary, you may need to have it done more than once to get an accurate reading. Ultrasound imaging is also used to estimate the size of your prostate gland. In addition, it can detect problems such as a kidney obstruction, stones in your kidneys or prostate, or a tumor.

### Urodynamic studies

If your doctor suspects that your symptoms may be related to a bladder problem rather than BPH, he or she may recommend tests to measure bladder pressure and function.

These tests are done by threading a small catheter through the urethra and into the bladder. Bladder pressure is measured during urination. Water also is injected into your bladder to measure internal bladder pressure and to determine how effectively your bladder contracts.

### Cystoscopy

This procedure involves a thin, flexible tube containing a lens with a light system (cystoscope) that's inserted into the urethra. It allows your doctor to see inside the urethra — including the part that goes through the prostate — and the bladder. The procedure can detect problems such as enlargement of the prostate, obstruction of the urethra or bladder neck, an anatomic abnormality, or the development of stones in your bladder.

### Intravenous pyelogram

An intravenous pyelogram (PI-uh-lo-gram ) is an X-ray image of the urinary tract, used to help detect an obstruction or abnormality. Dye is injected into a vein and an X-ray taken of your kidneys, bladder and the tubes that connect your kidneys to your bladder (ureters). The dye makes it possible to identify a blockage. Because of newer imaging techniques and risk of an allergic reaction to the dye, this procedure is used less often today.

## Answers to your questions

*Are the tests used to diagnose BPH painful?*
Most aren't painful. But you may experience mild discomfort.
Sometimes a local anesthetic is used to minimize any pain.
Advances in flexible cystoscopy have made this procedure — done
in your doctor's office — much easier to tolerate.

*Do men with larger prostates have more severe symptoms?*
No. This is a common misconception. You can have a very large
prostate gland with few or no symptoms, or a small gland with
severe symptoms. That's because BPH results from growth in the
center portion of the prostate, not the outside. Although it may
squeeze inside tissues, the growth doesn't always affect the overall
dimensions of the gland.

*Does BPH increase my odds of having cancer?*
No evidence exists that BPH increases your risk of prostate
cancer. The two conditions appear to develop independently
of each other.

*I've had several bladder infections in recent months. Could these be
related to BPH?*
There may be a relationship. BPH sometimes prevents a man from
completely emptying his bladder, and this can lead to infection.
Talk with your doctor about it and about the value of having testing done that can determine the amount of urine left behind in
your bladder after you urinate.

*If I'm diagnosed with BPH, do I have to have surgery?*
If your symptoms are mild and aren't much of a bother, you and
your doctor may chose to do nothing for the time being and engage
in watchful waiting as an approach. If your symptoms become
worse, it may be helpful to consider either medication or a minimally invasive procedure, to provide relief. See Chapter 5 for
details on treating BPH.

*My father has BPH. Does that mean I'll get it, too?*
Not necessarily. But because BPH does tend to run in families, your risk is greater than is someone's from a family in which BPH hasn't been diagnosed.

# Treating benign prostatic hyperplasia

D o you avoid social events so that you won't have to worry about long lines to the bathroom? Are you tired in the morning from getting up during the night to use the bathroom? Are you no longer wearing light-colored pants for fear of noticeable dribbling? These are common ways benign prostatic hyperplasia (BPH) can interfere with your life.

Many men would rather put up with the inconveniences of BPH than treat it. But if your symptoms have reached the point where they're affecting your quality of life, it may be time to see a doctor. Treatment for BPH comes in various forms.

## Watchful waiting

If your symptoms are mild — getting up to urinate once or twice during the night, for example — and you're not bothered by them, you and your doctor may decide that watchful waiting is appropriate. Your doctor may periodically evaluate your condition to see if it improves, stays the same or gets worse.

The advantage of watchful waiting is that you don't have to undergo any invasive treatment. Your treatment usually doesn't cost you anything beyond the usual fees for your physical examination and perhaps some tests. The risk you take with this approach is that your condition could worsen drastically or other problems may develop, such as an infection. But this is uncommon.

**While you wait**

Some simple lifestyle changes can often help control symptoms of BPH and prevent your condition from worsening.

**Limit beverages.** Stop drinking water and other beverages a few hours before bedtime to reduce your need to go to the bathroom.

**Empty your bladder.** Try to urinate all that you can each time you go to the bathroom.

**Limit alcohol.** Alcohol increases urine production and may cause congestion in the prostate gland.

**Be careful with over-the-counter decongestants.** They can cause the band of muscle that controls urine flow from your urethra (urethral sphincter) to tighten, making urination more difficult.

**Keep active.** Inactivity causes you to retain urine. Even a small amount of exercise can reduce urinary problems caused by BPH.

**Stay warm.** Cold weather can lead to urine retention.

## Medication

Drug therapy is the most common method for controlling moderate symptoms of BPH. Medication is also an option for men with mild BPH whose symptoms are annoying or for men who decide against watchful waiting.

There are two types of medications for BPH.

### Alpha blockers

These drugs were originally developed to treat high blood pressure, but they're also beneficial for other conditions, including BPH. They relax your urethral sphincter muscle, making it easier to urinate. The Food and Drug Administration has approved three alpha blockers for BPH:

- Terazosin (Hytrin)
- Doxazosin (Cardura)
- Tamsulosin (Flomax)

Alpha blockers are effective in about two-thirds of men who take them. The drugs also work quickly. Within just one or two days, most men notice an increase in urinary flow and a decrease in how often they need to urinate, particularly at night.

Doctors still are uncertain about the long-term benefits and risks of alpha blockers. However, the drugs appear to be safe. Side effects can include headaches or feeling dizzy, lightheaded or tired. For this reason, it's best to take the medication before bedtime. Some men also report feeling faint when standing too quickly, due to low blood pressure (orthostatic hypotension). To reduce your risk of these side effects, your doctor may start you out with a low dose of medication and gradually increase the dosage.

Tamsulosin may cause less dizziness. You also don't need to gradually increase its dosage. As a result, its benefits tend to be more noticeable and occur more quickly. Abnormal ejaculation can occur in men who take tamsulosin. However, adjusting the dosage may remedy the problem.

### Finasteride and dutasteride

Finasteride (Proscar) and dutasteride (Avodart) relieve BPH symptoms in a totally different manner. Instead of relaxing your pelvic muscles, they shrink your prostate gland. For some men with large prostates, these drugs may produce a noticeable improvement in symptoms. They're generally not effective, though, if you have a slightly enlarged or normal-sized prostate.

Finasteride takes a longer time to work than does dutasteride. You may notice some improvement in urinary flow after three months, but for complete results generally it takes up to a year. A small percentage of men who take finasteride experience impotence, decreased libido and reduced semen release during ejaculation. But in most men, finasteride produces only slight side effects.

Combining an alpha blocker with finasteride has shown more promise in reducing the progression of BPH than has using either drug separately. The Medical Therapy of Prostatic Symptoms (MTOPS) trial, published in 2002, found that men taking both the alpha blocker doxazosin (Cardura) and finasteride reduced their risk of BPH progression by 67 percent. Meanwhile, those who took the alpha blocker doxazosin alone reduced their risk by 39 percent and those who took finasteride alone cut their risk by 34 percent.

Finasteride recently has been shown to prevent or delay the onset of prostate cancer in men 55 years and older.

## Surgery

At one time, surgery was the most common treatment for BPH. But because of increased use of medications and the development of other less invasive therapies, surgery is on the decline. Today, it's used mainly when drug therapy fails to offer relief or if you have complicating factors, such as:

- Retention of urine
- Bleeding through the urethra
- Stones in the bladder

Surgery is the most effective of all therapies for relieving symptoms of BPH. It's the gold standard by which all other treatments are judged. However, it's also the most likely to produce postoperative problems. These include a small risk of impotence, a very small risk of uncontrolled urine leakage and risk of constricture of the urethra.

Fortunately, most men experience few problems. Among people with certain health conditions, such as uncontrolled diabetes, cirrhosis of the liver, any major psychiatric disorder, or serious lung, kidney or heart conditions, surgery isn't usually recommended.

There are three types of surgery for BPH.

### TURP

Transurethral resection of the prostate (TURP) is the most common of all prostate surgeries done to treat BPH.

During the procedure, you're placed under general anesthesia or anesthetized from the waist down with a spinal block. A surgeon threads a narrow instrument (resectoscope) into the urethra and uses small cutting tools contained in the resectoscope to scrape away excess prostate tissue (see illustration on page 49). You can expect to stay in the hospital for one to three days after this surgery. During recovery you'll have a urinary catheter for a few days.

TURP is effective and relieves symptoms quickly. Most men experience a stronger urine flow within a few days. You can expect some blood or small blood clots to appear in your urine afterward. Before you leave the hospital you should be able to urinate on your own. At first you may feel some pain or a sense of urgency when urine passes over the surgical area. This discomfort should gradually improve.

In a few cases, TURP can cause impotence and loss of bladder control. These conditions are generally only temporary. Pelvic floor muscle exercises (Kegel exercises) will often help restore bladder control (see "Strengthening your pelvic floor muscles" on page 109). Normal sexual function often returns within a few weeks to months. However, it can take up to a year for full recovery.

Another more common side effect of this surgery is dry climax (retrograde ejaculation). In this condition, semen flows backward into your bladder during orgasm instead of out through the penis, causing infertility. TURP may also produce scarring and narrowing in the urethra. This often can be remedied by a simple stretching procedure done on an outpatient basis.

Between 10 percent and 20 percent of men who have TURP need surgery again within 10 to 15 years because the prostate tissue grows back.

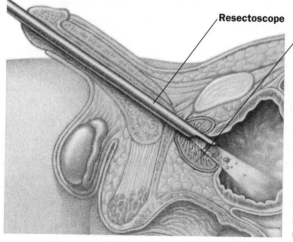

Resectoscope

Prostate gland enlarged by BPH

Transurethral resection of the prostate (TURP) is the most common surgery for benign prostatic hyperplasia (BPH). A thin instrument (resectoscope) is threaded through the urethra to where it's surrounded by the prostate. Tiny cutting tools on the resectoscope scrape away excess prostate tissue, improving urine flow.

## TUIP

Transurethral incision of the prostate (TUIP) is an option if you have a moderately enlarged or small prostate gland. It's also an option for men who aren't good candidates for more invasive surgery for health reasons or because they don't want to risk sterility from retrograde ejaculation.

Like TURP, TUIP involves special instruments that are inserted through the urethra. But instead of removing prostate tissue, the surgeon makes one or two small cuts in the prostate gland. The cuts help enlarge the opening of the urethra, making it easier to urinate.

The procedure produces less risk of complications than do other kinds of surgery, and it doesn't require an overnight hospital stay. However, TUIP is less effective and it often needs to be repeated. Some men experience only a small improvement in urinary flow.

### Open prostatectomy

The most common type of open prostatectomy is radical prostatectomy to remove a cancerous prostate gland. It involves removing the entire gland. During a partial prostatectomy for the treatment of BPH, only the inner portion of the gland is removed, leaving the outer portion intact.

This type of surgery is generally performed only if you have an excessively large prostate, you have bladder damage or you have other complicating factors, such as stones in your bladder. It's called open prostatectomy because the surgeon makes an incision in your lower abdomen to reach the prostate, rather than going up through the urethra.

Open prostatectomy is the most effective therapy for relieving BPH. Improvement of symptoms has been reported by 98 percent of men who underwent the procedure. However, open prostatectomy also poses the greatest risk of side effects. Complications of the procedure are similar to those of TURP, but their effects may be more pronounced. The procedure usually requires a hospital stay of about four to five days.

### Recovering from surgery

Depending on the type of surgery you have, it may take a couple of weeks to several months for a full recovery. During this time, avoid activities that involve lifting, jarring to your pelvic area, such as from operating heavy equipment or riding a bicycle, and overly straining of your lower abdominal muscles, such as during a bowel movement.

To prevent constipation, eat plenty of high-fiber foods, such as fruits, vegetables and grains. Fiber softens stool and makes it easier to pass. Drinking eight glasses of water daily also helps cleanse your urinary tract and promote healing.

# Heat, or minimally invasive, therapies

Heat therapies — also called thermal therapies — are less invasive treatments than TURP, TUIP and open prostatectomy surgery. Minimally invasive therapies use various types of energy — including microwave, radiofrequency and laser — to create heat that destroys excessive prostate tissue. The basic principle at work is to deliver enough heat for enough time to cause prostate cell death. These treatments may be more effective than medication for moderate to severe symptoms, and they don't produce as many side effects as does surgery. There are several types of heat therapies.

### Microwave therapy

Transurethral microwave therapy (TUMT) is a computer-controlled application of microwave energy to heat and destroy the inner portion of an enlarged prostate.

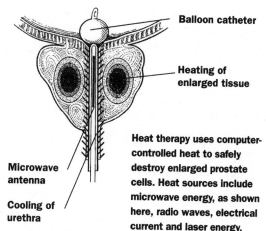

**Balloon catheter**

**Heating of enlarged tissue**

**Microwave antenna**

**Cooling of urethra**

Heat therapy uses computer-controlled heat to safely destroy enlarged prostate cells. Heat sources include microwave energy, as shown here, radio waves, electrical current and laser energy.

During the procedure, a machine emits microwave energy through a urinary catheter. The catheter includes a tiny internal microwave antenna to deliver a dose of microwave energy that heats the enlarged cells and destroys them. Cool water circulates around the tip and sides of the antenna during the procedure to protect the urethra from the heat.

A local anesthetic helps control pain. You may feel some heat in the prostate and bladder area. You may also have a strong desire to urinate and may experience bladder spasms. These responses are usually well tolerated and disappear after the treatment is finished. You can go home after TUMT when you're urinating satisfactorily — usually the same day of your treatment. About 30 percent of men need to wear a urinary catheter for several days to a week and sometimes longer after the procedure.

Unlike TURP, it may take several weeks before you begin to see a noticeable improvement in your symptoms. The long-term effectiveness of the procedure is also uncertain. One study found that about 60 percent of men were satisfied with the results of their TUMT treatment after one year, but only 23 percent of the men were satisfied four years later. Two-thirds of them had sought supplementary BPH treatment. Those who seem to respond best over time are men whose initial symptoms are mild, or who've had success with BPH medications and wish to be off them.

It's normal to have urgency, frequent urination and small amounts of blood in your urine during recovery. You may also experience a change in the amount of semen you ejaculate. However, unlike more invasive surgery, TUMT generally doesn't produce impotence, incontinence or retrograde ejaculation.

The procedure isn't recommended if you have a penile prosthesis or any metal implants in your penis.

### Radiofrequency therapy

Transurethral needle ablation (TUNA) uses the energy of high-frequency radio waves to heat and destroy tissue. This energy is delivered directly to the prostate by two needles that are guided into the prostate by a special catheter called a cystoscope. The needles are inserted into the prostate by precisely maneuvering the cystoscope.

TUNA typically is less effective than traditional surgery but similar to TUMT in reducing symptoms and improving urine flow. This form of heat energy gives your doctor the advantage of tailoring treatment to unusual prostate configurations. Its long-term effectiveness isn't fully known, and it isn't approved for use in men with large prostates.

The procedure, however, doesn't produce incontinence or impotence. Side effects may include urine retention, blood in your urine, painful urination and a small risk of retrograde ejaculation.

### Electrovaporization

Transurethral electrovaporization of the prostate (TUVP) is a modification of the TURP procedure that provides nearly bloodless removal of prostate tissue, along with a shorter hospital stay and less catheterization time. However, the time for TUVP treatment may be longer than for TURP because it takes longer to vaporize prostate tissue than to cut it.

It involves a special metal instrument that emits a high-frequency electrical current to vaporize excess tissue, while sealing off the tissue to prevent bleeding.

TUVP may be as effective as TURP, without the high cost and with fewer complications. Because this type of surgery is technically simpler and causes less bleeding, it's useful for men at higher risk of complications, including those taking blood-thinning medication.

As with other minimally invasive treatments, its long-term benefits aren't yet known.

### Laser therapies

Laser therapies are performed similarly to other heat therapies, but they use laser light energy instead of microwave energy, radio waves or electrical current to produce heat. They generally don't cause impotence or prolonged incontinence. However, some laser procedures require lengthy use of a catheter.

There are several types of lasers used to treat enlarged prostates. They include the neodymium:yttrium-aluminum-garnet (Nd:YAG), KTP, holmium:YAG and diode lasers.

**TUEP.** Transurethral evaporation of the prostate (TUEP) is similar to electrovaporization. The difference is that your doctor uses laser energy instead of electrical current to destroy prostate tissue. The procedure is generally safe and causes limited bleeding. It's often effective, with noticeable improvement in urine flow soon after the procedure.

**VLAP.** Visual laser ablation of the prostate (VLAP) involves applying enough laser energy to dry up and destroy excess prostate cells, which you eventually eliminate over several weeks to months. One major drawback lessens its appeal: Because of swelling and prolonged sloughing off of the dead tissue, you're likely to retain urine for several days and will need to wear a catheter. You may also experience a burning sensation for days to weeks during urination.

## Building a better laser

One of the biggest drawbacks to laser therapy is the need for wearing a catheter for a prolonged period after treatment. Newer, high-energy types of lasers are helping solve this problem.

The newer lasers work by destroying excess prostate tissue, either by cutting it out or by vaporizing it. This allows immediate removal of obstructive tissue, so you need a catheter for only 24 hours at most. Technologies being evaluated include the KTP, the photoselective vaporization of the prostate (PVP), the holmium:YAG and the holmium laser enucleation of the prostate (HoLEP) lasers. Mayo Clinic urologists have pioneered the use of the KTP laser with continued success.

The goal is to combine the advantages of laser therapy — safety and limited bleeding — with immediate improvement in urinary flow that comes with more invasive surgery.

**Interstitial laser therapy.** This procedure directs laser energy deeper inside the prostate gland rather than at the urethral surface. It moderately increases the urinary flow rate and reduces the size of the prostate. It also seems to work well for men with large prostate glands.

Because of substantial tissue inflammation after treatment, you may need to use a catheter for up to three weeks. Interstitial laser therapy doesn't cause any blood loss and is a good option if you can't have surgery.

### Prostatic stents

With this treatment, a tiny coated metal coil is inserted into your urethra to widen and hold open the urethral portion of the prostate gland. Tissue grows over the stent to hold it in place.

One advantage of the procedure is that it takes only 10 to 15 minutes and doesn't require anesthesia. It also produces little or no bleeding and doesn't require a catheter. However, some studies show that about 23 percent of men with stents have them removed because of poor placement or complications.

Some men find that the stents don't improve their symptoms, and others experience irritation when urinating or have urinary tract infections.

These complications, along with potential difficulties in removing the stents when they cause problems, have reduced their use. Stents are generally recommended for men troubled by urine retention who want to be catheter-free and who can't tolerate other minimally invasive procedures because of age or illness.

---

## A BPH shot?

Because benign prostatic hyperplasia (BPH) is such a common problem, new therapies to treat it are being explored. Transurethral injection of various agents including alcohol, drugs or enzymes may play a role in future treatment. By way of a catheter, a combination of substances is injected into the prostate to dissolve excess tissue. Laboratory studies and preliminary studies in men suggest that the procedure is safe and effective. Mayo Clinic is among those institutions studying this form of injection treatment.

Researchers also are studying the effects of injecting high-concentration salt solutions into enlarged prostates. In an effort to dilute the salt solution, prostate cells absorb additional water. The cells take in so much water that they rupture and die.

---

## Weighing your options

With so many options to choose from, deciding on the best way to treat BPH can be difficult. Each treatment may improve your symptoms, but in different ways. Each also has its advantages and disadvantages. The question becomes which one will best meet your needs with the fewest side effects. As you and your doctor plan your treatment strategy, consider these important factors:

### Severity of your symptoms

If your symptoms don't bother you and your condition isn't causing any other problems, you can probably wait to see if your symptoms improve or worsen. On the other hand, if you have severe symptoms, organ damage or complicating factors, such as frequent urinary infections, bleeding or bladder stones, you may need surgery.

Treatment for anything in between depends on your personal preference. Will you settle for a small improvement in symptoms, or are you hoping for something more noticeable? Do you want immediate relief or can you wait? Are you willing to take medication daily? Will you tolerate some side effects?

### Size of your gland
Some treatments are best suited for large prostates (40 grams and larger). Others are more effective for smaller to moderately sized prostates. Therapies best suited for large prostates include:
- Finasteride (Proscar) or dutasteride (Avodart)
- Transurethral resection of the prostate (TURP)
- Open prostatectomy
- Transurethral microwave therapy (TUMT)
- Laser therapy

Treatments more appropriate for small to moderately sized prostates include:
- Alpha blockers
- Transurethral incision of the prostate (TUIP)
- Transurethral needle ablation (TUNA)
- Transurethral electrovaporization of the prostate (TUVP)
- Laser therapy

### Your age
The best treatment for a man in his 50s may not be the best for a man in his 80s. If you're younger, you may want a treatment that provides long-term benefits. If you're older, immediate benefits may be more important than long-term effects. In addition, younger men often recover more quickly from surgery and other invasive procedures than do men in their 70s or 80s.

### Your health
If you have other health conditions, you may not be a good candidate for surgery or recover as quickly. Surgery generally isn't

recommended if you have:
- Uncontrolled diabetes
- Cirrhosis of the liver
- Serious lung, kidney or heart disease
- A major psychiatric disorder

Some people aren't good candidates for medication because of intolerance to a specific drug or certain kinds of medication.

### Your fertility

If you want to father children, you'll want to avoid therapies that could cause infertility. TURP, TUIP, open prostatectomy and laser therapy can lead to retrograde ejaculation, in which semen backs up into your bladder instead of ejaculating from your penis. The risk of retrograde ejaculation varies depending on the procedure. With TURP, the risk is about 70 percent. TUIP carries about a 40-percent risk, and with open prostatectomy, the risk is about 80 percent. Less often, TUNA, interstitial laser therapy and alpha blockers also can cause retrograde ejaculation. Unlike impotence, which may be temporary, retrograde ejaculation is usually permanent.

### Your sexuality

Surgery can damage nerves or blood vessels located next to the prostate gland, causing impotence. Your odds of experiencing impotence after TURP are about 14 percent. Often, however, normal sexual function, including the ability to have an erection and an orgasm, returns after a few months.

Impotence — even for a short time — is a concern for many men. Discuss this issue with your doctor before surgery.

### Benefits vs. risks

Do the benefits of the procedure you're considering outweigh the risks? (See "A brief comparison" on page 59.)

TURP is the most common treatment for BPH, in large part because it has been used for years and doctors know its long-term effects. But it also poses some risks. In addition to impotence and retrograde ejaculation, TURP is associated with urinary tract infection in about 16 percent of men and incontinence in about 1 percent.

Open prostatectomy has greater benefits and risks, but because it's more invasive, it's less commonly used.

Minimally invasive therapies appear to be effective, and they generally produce fewer side effects. Relief from symptoms typically occurs more slowly with minimally invasive therapies than with surgery. And because some of these therapies are still fairly new, their long-term benefits aren't fully known.

As for medication, alpha blockers, finasteride and dutasteride appear to offer long-term benefits, especially when used in combination. However, the drugs can cause side effects in some men.

### Expertise of your doctor

You want to select a therapy in which your doctor has considerable knowledge. Generally, the more experience your doctor has with the therapy, the less risk of side effects and the greater your odds for noticeable improvement.

### Recovery time

Recovery varies with the treatment. If you choose medication, you don't have to worry about being laid up or missing work.

Heat therapy is often performed on an outpatient basis. However, depending on the procedure, your doctor, and how quickly you're able to urinate on your own, you may need to stay in the hospital overnight. Heat therapy ordinarily requires only a few days' recovery time. An exception is laser therapy. Some older laser procedures require that you wear a catheter for up to three weeks. Newer techniques often require use of a catheter for only 24 hours.

Surgery for BPH requires a hospital stay. Plan for a two- to five-day stay if you have open prostatectomy. TURP and TUIP may mean a stay of one to three days in the hospital. In some cases, TUIP is done on an outpatient basis.

If you have an open prostatectomy, you may need to take up to a month off from work. For up to two months, you'll also need to avoid heavy lifting, jarring to your lower pelvic area, or straining of your lower abdominal muscles.

# A brief comparison

| Treatment | Advantages | Disadvantages |
|---|---|---|
| ***Medical***<br>**Watchful waiting** | Causes no side effects or complications. | Symptoms could become more severe. |
| **Alpha blockers** | Help three out of four men. Work quickly. | Can cause flu-like symptoms and dizziness. Long-term effects not fully known. |
| **Finasteride and dutasteride** | Cause few side effects. | Most effective with large prostates. Work slowly. |
| ***Minimally invasive***<br>**Transurethral microwave therapy (TUMT)** | Generally effective. Fewer side effects than TURP. An outpatient procedure. | Results can take several weeks. Long-term effects uncertain. |
| **Transurethral needle ablation (TUNA)** | Generally effective. Causes few side effects. An outpatient procedure. | Less effective with larger prostates. Results take time. Long-term effects un-known. |
| **Transurethral electrovaporization of the prostate (TUVP)** | Similar in effectiveness to TURP. Few side effects. Doesn't cause blood loss. | One to two day hospital stay. Long-term effects unknown. |
| **Laser therapy (TUEP, VLAP, others)** | As effective as TURP. Newer lasers cause minimal side effects. Outpatient procedure. | Some older forms of treatment can require lengthy use of a catheter. |
| **Stents** | Don't require surgery. Quick procedure. Only for men too ill to have surgery. | Often not effective. Can cause bothersome side effects. |
| ***Surgery***<br>**Transurethral resection of the prostate (TURP)** | Most common form of surgery. Effective and provides immediate results. | One to three day hospital stay. Small risk of impotence and incontinence. Can cause retrograde ejaculation. |
| **Transurethral incision of the prostate (TUIP)** | An outpatient procedure. Fewer side effects. Doesn't cause retrograde ejaculation. | Not as effective as TURP. Less effective in large prostates. |
| **Open prostatectomy** | Most effective therapy. Only for large prostates. | Greatest risk of side effects. Longer hospital stay. |

## Answers to your questions

*Can treatment for BPH reduce my risk of getting cancer?*
It may, depending on the treatment. A recent study showed that taking the drug finasteride prevented or delayed the onset of prostate cancer by 25 percent in men age 55 and older. However, the same study showed that finasteride contributed to increased sexual side effects and slightly raised the risk of developing higher-grade prostate cancer.

Other BPH treatments don't reduce the risk of prostate cancer, with the exception of complete prostate removal. Even if you're being treated for BPH, you still need to continue regular prostate exams to screen for cancer. Some treatments for BPH, however, can identify cancer in its early stages. For example, unsuspected cancer is found during TURP in about 10 percent to 15 percent of men.

*Is Proscar the same drug used for hair growth?*
Yes. Finasteride is used to treat both BPH and hair loss. The only difference is the dose. Proscar, for BPH, comes in a 5-milligram (mg) tablet. Propecia, for hair growth, comes in a 1-mg tablet.

*If the first option I choose doesn't work, can I try another?*
Absolutely. Conservative options, such as medication, are often the first choice of many men and their doctors. If conservative options don't produce satisfactory results, then you can move on to an invasive procedure.

*Should I get a second opinion before deciding on a treatment?*
Not necessarily. It depends on the confidence you have in your doctor and the therapeutic option that you choose. If you select a more conservative treatment, such as medication, or a minimally invasive therapy, your doctor has adequate experience with the therapy, and you feel comfortable with the decision, a second opinion may not be necessary. If you don't feel comfortable with your doctor's recommendation, it might be a good idea to consult another doctor.

# Part 3

*Prostate cancer*

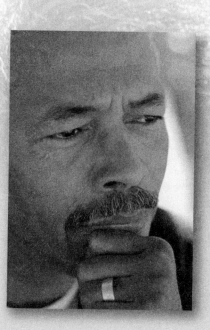

## Chapter 6

# *Learning you have cancer*

Prostate cancer is the most commonly diagnosed life-threatening cancer in men in the United States. It's the second-leading cause of cancer deaths in American men — lung cancer is the leading cause. Each year, about 220,000 new cases of prostate cancer are diagnosed. It's estimated that by age 50, up to one in three men have some cancerous cells in the prostate gland. By age 75, the rate increases to about three in four. In many of these cases, the cancer produces no signs or symptoms and is called latent. In other cases, the cancer does produce signs and symptoms, but they're not serious threats to your health. In such instances, the cancer is considered indolent. As you age, your risk of prostate cancer increases. The average age at diagnosis of prostate cancer is 72.

## What exactly is cancer?

Cancer, simply put, is a group of abnormal cells that grow more rapidly than do normal cells and don't die off. Your body continuously produces new cells that live only a short time before being replaced by fresh cells. Skin cells, for example, live just a few weeks. But microscopic cancer cells grow into small nodules or pea-sized collections that continue to grow, becoming more densely packed and hard.

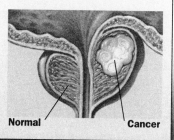

Normal | Cancer

# Estimated new cancer cases and deaths — 2003*

## Cancer cases by site and sex

### Men

| Prostate | 220,900 |
| Lung & bronchus | 91,800 |
| Colon & rectum | 72,800 |
| Urinary bladder | 42,200 |
| Non-Hodgkin's lymphoma | 28,300 |
| Skin (melanoma) | 29,900 |
| Oral cavity | 18,200 |
| Kidney | 19,500 |
| Leukemia | 17,900 |
| Pancreas | 14,900 |
| All cancers | 675,300 |

### Women

| Breast | 211,300 |
| Lung & bronchus | 80,100 |
| Colon & rectum | 74,700 |
| Uterine corpus | 40,100 |
| Ovary | 25,400 |
| Non-Hodgkin's lymphoma | 25,100 |
| Skin (melanoma) | 24,300 |
| Urinary bladder | 15,200 |
| Pancreas | 15,800 |
| Thyroid | 16,300 |
| All cancers | 658,800 |

## Cancer deaths by site and sex

### Men

| Lung & bronchus | 88,400 |
| Prostate | 28,900 |
| Colon & rectum | 28,300 |
| Pancreas | 14,700 |
| Non-Hodgkin's lymphoma | 12,200 |
| Leukemia | 12,100 |
| Esophagus | 9,900 |
| Liver | 9,200 |
| Urinary bladder | 8,600 |
| Stomach | 7,000 |
| All cancers | 285,900 |

### Women

| Lung & bronchus | 68,800 |
| Breast | 39,800 |
| Colon & rectum | 28,800 |
| Pancreas | 15,300 |
| Ovary | 14,300 |
| Non-Hodgkin's lymphoma | 11,200 |
| Leukemia | 9,800 |
| Uterine corpus | 6,800 |
| Brain | 5,800 |
| Stomach | 5,100 |
| All cancers | 270,600 |

*Excluding basal and squamous cell skin cancers and *in situ* carcinomas, except urinary bladder cancer.

Source: American Cancer Society

On average, an American man has about a 16-percent risk of being diagnosed with prostate cancer, about an 8-percent chance the cancer will cause significant symptoms, and about a 3-percent risk of dying of the disease.

Typically, prostate cancer grows slowly and remains confined to the prostate gland, where it doesn't cause serious harm. But not all cancers act the same. Some forms of prostate cancer can be aggressive, and these cancers can quickly spread to other parts of the body.

What causes prostate cancer and why some types behave differently are unknown. Research suggests a combination of factors may play a role, including family history, ethnicity, hormones, diet and environment (see "Are you at risk?" on page 8).

However, this much is clear. Most men with prostate cancer that's detected while the cancer is still confined to the prostate gland can be cured. It's after the cancer has spread to nearby organs that treating the disease becomes more difficult — but not impossible. The goal of early treatment is both to stop prostate cancer before it spreads and to preserve quality of life, which can be negatively affected by a cancer that has spread.

## Signs and symptoms that may signal cancer

The problem with prostate cancer is that it often doesn't produce any signs or symptoms in its early stages, when it's the easiest to treat. But the good news is that — at least in part due to better screening methods and increased awareness of the need for screening — approximately 75 percent of prostate cancers are now diagnosed in the first round of screening, before they've spread beyond the prostate.

When symptoms of advanced prostate cancer do develop, they may be much like those you would experience with benign prostatic hyperplasia (BPH). You may also feel in your lower pelvic area a dull pain that doesn't subside. Signs and symptoms may include:

- A sudden need to urinate
- Difficulty starting to urinate
- Pain during urination
- Weak urine flow and dribbling
- Starting and stopping of your urine flow

- A sensation that your bladder isn't empty
- Frequent urination at night
- Blood in your urine
- Painful ejaculation
- General pain in the lower back, hips or upper thighs
- Loss of appetite and weight

Although these signs and symptoms aren't always indicative of prostate cancer, they do call for evaluation by your doctor.

## How prostate cancer is diagnosed

A digital rectal examination and the prostate-specific antigen (PSA) test are usually the first steps in diagnosing prostate cancer. If the results of one or both tests are abnormal and your doctor suspects cancer, he or she may have you undergo a biopsy. Analyzing small tissue samples from the gland is the most effective way to tell if you have prostate cancer.

To do a biopsy, your doctor will insert an ultrasound probe into your rectum. Guided by images from the probe identifying suspect areas, your doctor directs a fine, hollow needle at various parts of the prostate gland. Called a biopsy gun, this needle is powered by a spring that instantly propels and retrieves very thin sections of tissue.

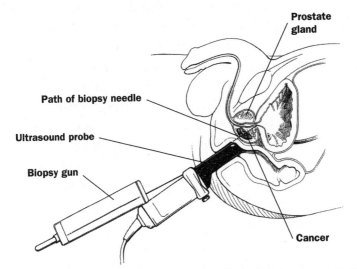

During a biopsy, a biopsy gun quickly projects a thin needle into suspect areas of the prostate gland and small sections of tissue are retrieved for analysis.

Occasionally, the biopsy needle is inserted into your prostate through the perineum, the area between the anus and the scrotum. More often, it's directed alongside the ultrasound probe and inserted through the rectum.

During the biopsy, your doctor may take as many as 10 to 12 sections of tissue from different areas of your prostate gland. Most of the samples are taken from the outer area of your gland (peripheral zone), where most cancers start. Sometimes, samples are taken from the inner portion of the gland (transitional zone).

A prostate biopsy is commonly performed using local anesthesia that reduces or eliminates the pain and discomfort once associated with this procedure. Most men have virtually no pain during the procedure and usually don't require pain medication afterward.

You'll be given an enema. This reduces the risk of infection from digestive bacteria that might otherwise enter the needle incision. Antibiotics taken before and after the biopsy also further reduce the possibility of infection.

Common side effects of a biopsy include a small amount of rectal bleeding and blood in your urine for one to two days. Blood may appear in your semen (hematospermia), giving it a pink tint, for weeks to months afterward.

The tissue samples taken from your prostate are sent to a pathologist who specializes in diagnosing cancer and other tissue abnormalities. From the samples, the pathologist can tell if it's cancer and how aggressive the cancer is.

The biopsy samples can also identify specific cells that put you at significant risk of having cancer in the future. Known as prostatic intraepithelial neoplasia (PIN), these abnormal cells are in the early stage of becoming cancerous. If PIN is found, your doctor may recommend additional biopsies. For men with more severe (high-grade) PIN, there's a 30-percent to 50-percent chance of finding prostate cancer on a later biopsy. If you have high-grade PIN, your doctor may closely monitor your PSA levels and recommend another biopsy in six months.

## Grading the cancer

When a biopsy confirms the presence of cancer, the next step, called grading, is done to determine if it's a slow- or fast-growing form. A pathologist studies your prostate tissue samples on a series of slides under a microscope, comparing the cancer cells with healthy prostate cells. The more the cancer cells differ from the healthy cells, the more aggressive the cancer and the more likely it is to spread quickly.

Throughout the samples, cancer cells may vary in shape and size. Some cells may be aggressive, others not. The pathologist identifies the two most prominent types of cancer cells when assigning a grade.

Prostate cancer cells are graded on several kinds of scales. The most common scale runs from 1 to 5, with 1 being the least aggressive form of cancer. The scale is named after pathologist Donald Gleason, M.D., who devised it.

**Grade 1.** Cancer cells are small, shaped much alike and are evenly spaced, similar to healthy cells.

**Grade 2.** Cancer cells are more varied in size and shape, and more loosely scattered.

**Grade 3.** Cancer cells are even more varied in size and shape, with some cells fused together into large, oddly shaped clumps that are scattered about.

**Grade 4.** Many cancer cells are fused into masses that are scattered haphazardly and are invading nearby tissue.

**Grade 5.** Most cancer cells have gathered into large, scattered masses that have invaded nearby tissues and organs.

The two most numerous types of cancer cells in your biopsy each get one of these five grades. For example, your primary grade of cancer could be a 3, while your secondary grade of cancer could be a 4. These two numbers are added together to determine a total Gleason score — in this case, 7. The lower the score the better. Scores between 2 and 4 likely mean the cancer is slow-growing. Scores in the middle — 5 and 6 — can mean the cancer is slow- or fast-growing, depending on a variety of factors, including how long you've had the cancer. A score of 7 indicates a more aggressive cancer, and scores at the high end of the scale, from 8 to 10, mean the cancer is fast-growing.

A study published in 1998 estimated what the risk was of dying of prostate cancer for men age 55 to 74 with localized disease who were treated conservatively, that is without surgery or radiation therapy. The researchers estimated that men with Gleason scores of 2 to 4 had a minimal risk — 4 percent to 7 percent — of dying of prostate cancer within 15 years of diagnosis. Men in the middle range with scores of 5 and 6 had a modest risk of dying — 6 percent to 11 percent for a score of 5, and 18 percent to 30 percent for a score of 6. Men with a score of 7 had a risk of 42 percent to 70 percent, and men with scores of 8 to 10 had a risk between 60 percent and 87 percent.

## Interpreting the grades

Studies suggest that with Gleason scores of 2 to 4, there's about a 12-percent chance that prostate cancer will have spread to lymph nodes in the pelvis. With Gleason scores of 5 to 7, there's about a 35-percent chance the cancer has spread, and with scores of 8 to 10, there's about a 61-percent chance the cancer has spread beyond the prostate gland to lymph nodes in the region.

## Has the cancer spread?

This determination is crucial because cancer confined to the prostate has a high cure rate. Once the cancer extends beyond the prostate, the survival rate declines. Further tests will help determine whether the cancer has spread. Depending on your doctor and your cancer, you may have one or more of the following tests.

### Ultrasound
Ultrasound may be used to measure the dimensions of your prostate gland in order to plan some treatment procedures. It's not necessary to use it in all cases.

### Bone scan
This is the most common test because it can show the spread of cancer to bone better than other procedures. However, a bone scan

isn't necessary in evaluating all cases, and it's generally not used when there's little reason to suspect the cancer has spread.

Beforehand, a harmless, low-grade radioactive solution is injected into your bloodstream. This is a tracer solution that the bone scan will pick up plainly in a full-body skeletal image. The solution travels throughout your body and attaches itself to areas of new bone growth that may stem from cancer or from fractures, arthritis or infections.

During the scan, you lie on an examination table beneath a scanner. An image of your skeleton is displayed on a monitor, with areas of rapid growth showing up as dark spots on the picture.

Interpreting the bone scan can be difficult in some people because the scan picks up more than cancer. However, doctors know that prostate cancer tends to spread first to bones near the prostate, such as the hips and lower spine. In addition, isolated spots in one area are more typical of cancer than are corresponding spots on both sides of the body, such as those indicating arthritis in your right and left hips.

### Chest X-ray

An X-ray film can show if the cancer has spread to your lungs. Though less than 5 percent of prostate cancer spreads this far, studies have shown that lung cancer has developed in about 50 percent of people with advanced prostate cancer.

### CT scan

A computerized tomography (CT) scan produces three-dimensional, cross-sectional images of your body tissues that are stacked together on a computer screen, allowing a doctor to view specific parts of your body from any angle. A CT scan isn't necessary in every case. As with a bone scan, your doctor may decide to order a CT scan only if there's reason to suspect that the cancer has spread.

Before the CT scan, an iodine-based solution is injected into your bloodstream. This provides enhanced contrast to the X-ray images for clearer pictures. You may feel a temporary rush of heat as the solution spreads throughout your body, but you'll experience no pain. It's possible to do CT without the iodine if you're allergic to the solution, but the pictures won't be as clear.

Here's how CT works. You lie on a table that slowly glides through the middle of a large donut-shaped scanner. While you're lying down, the scanner takes a series of pictures showing different "slices" of tissue in the area of your prostate. The process may take up to 30 minutes.

A computer then stacks the image slices together to form a detailed picture of your prostate and the area surrounding it. In addition to cancer, a CT scan can identify enlarged lymph nodes. When cancer begins to spread, one of the first places it goes to is your lymph nodes. The lymph nodes trap and try to destroy abnormal cells, causing the nodes to swell and become overwhelmed by the cancer.

Unfortunately, CT can identify only lymph nodes that look abnormal, not those with microscopic levels of cancer. Your lymph nodes may be swollen for other reasons. Therefore, CT is most useful only when combined with other tests.

## MRI

Like CT, magnetic resonance imaging (MRI) produces a detailed, three-dimensional picture of your body. Its primary value in the diagnosis of prostate cancer is to detect the spread of cancer to lymph nodes and bone. In this way, it may assist in staging either localized or advanced prostate cancer.

Instead of using X-rays and dyes to generate the pictures, MRI uses magnetic and radio waves. A radiofrequency pulse passes through your body, generating a current that is picked up on a radiofrequency receiver and is then translated into a picture that looks much like a CT image.

During MRI, you lie inside a small, tube-shaped device for 30 to 45 minutes. It's not painful, but the machine makes noises, like those of a woodpecker, and some people get anxious when enclosed in the small space. If this might be a problem for you, a sedative beforehand can help calm you.

## Lymph node biopsy

The best way to determine if the cancer has spread to nearby lymph nodes is with a lymphadenectomy (lim-fad-uh-NEK-tuh-me). During this procedure, some of the nodes near the prostate are

# Prostate cancer staging

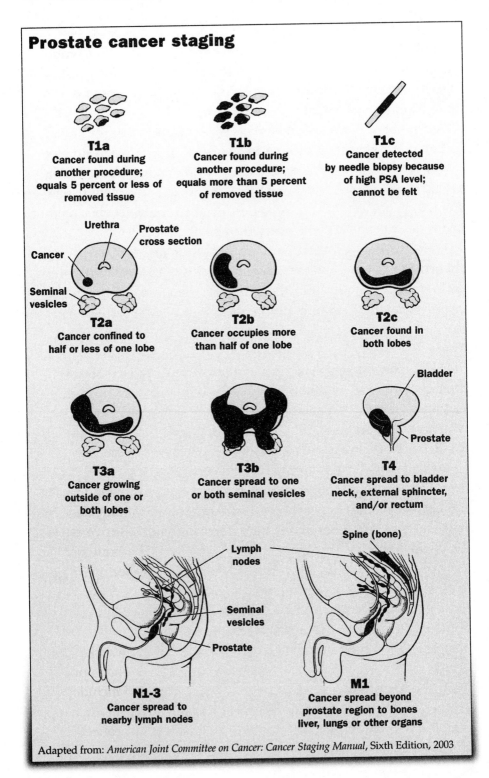

**T1a**
Cancer found during another procedure; equals 5 percent or less of removed tissue

**T1b**
Cancer found during another procedure; equals more than 5 percent of removed tissue

**T1c**
Cancer detected by needle biopsy because of high PSA level; cannot be felt

Urethra

Prostate cross section

Cancer

Seminal vesicles

**T2a**
Cancer confined to half or less of one lobe

**T2b**
Cancer occupies more than half of one lobe

**T2c**
Cancer found in both lobes

Bladder

Prostate

**T3a**
Cancer growing outside of one or both lobes

**T3b**
Cancer spread to one or both seminal vesicles

**T4**
Cancer spread to bladder neck, external sphincter, and/or rectum

Spine (bone)

Lymph nodes

Seminal vesicles

Prostate

**N1-3**
Cancer spread to nearby lymph nodes

**M1**
Cancer spread beyond prostate region to bones liver, lungs or other organs

Adapted from: *American Joint Committee on Cancer: Cancer Staging Manual*, Sixth Edition, 2003

removed and examined under a microscope. If other tests, such as a bone or CT scan, show that the cancer has spread, then a lymph-adenectomy usually isn't necessary. The procedure is most often used to confirm the results of tests indicating that the cancer is confined to the prostate.

There are two ways to remove lymph nodes:

**Laparoscopic surgery.** Following general anesthesia, a surgeon makes a couple of small incisions in your abdomen. Using a long surgical instrument that contains a tiny fiber-optic camera (laparoscope), your doctor removes lymph nodes from your pelvic area and sends them to a pathologist for analysis.

**Traditional surgery.** Once you've been anesthetized, a surgeon makes about a 3-inch incision between your navel and pubic area, and then locates and removes the lymph nodes through the incision. This method is most often done if your doctor is planning to do surgery to remove the prostate gland.

## Staging the cancer

Once all of your diagnostic tests are complete, your doctor will use the results of the tests to assign a stage to the cancer. This designation communicates to other health care personnel how advanced the cancer is.

Some men find staging information helpful in understanding the severity of their disease, and in discussing possible treatment options with their doctor. Other men find the information a little overwhelming. The important point is that if you have questions about your diagnosis or cancer stage, discuss them with your doctor.

Most doctors use one of two staging systems.

### TNM system

This is the most popular method in the United States for identifying the progression of cancer. When the pathologist sends your doctor a report that stages your cancer, the report will include three capital letters — T, N and M.

- T stands for tumor and signifies the extent of the cancer in, and adjacent to, the prostate gland.

---

**TNM stage groupings**

| | |
|---|---|
| **Stage I** | T1, N0, M0 |
| **Stage II** | T1-2, N0, M0 |
| **Stage III** | T3, N0, M0 |
| **Stage IV** | T4, N0, M0; Any T, N1-3, M0; Any T, any N, M1 |

Adapted from: *American Joint Committee on Cancer: Cancer Staging Manual*, Sixth Edition, 2003

---

- N stands for nodes (lymph nodes) and signifies whether the cancer has, or has not, spread to nearby lymph nodes.
- M stands for metastasis (muh-TAS-tuh-sis), the medical term for cancer that has spread to other tissues or organs, such as bone or the lungs.

The three letters are followed by a number and perhaps another letter in small type. The numbers range from 0 to 4 and represent the extent of the tumor. The small letters go from a to c and indicate location of the cancer.

Once the T, N and M results are known, the cancer is then assigned one of four stages based on the findings (see "TNM stage groupings" above).

**Stage I.** This signifies very early cancer that's confined to microscopic particles that can't be felt.

**Stage II.** The cancer can be felt, but it remains confined to the prostate gland.

**Stage III.** The cancer has spread beyond the prostate to the seminal vesicles or nearby bladder tissue.

**Stage IV.** This represents advanced cancer that has spread to lymph nodes, bones, lungs or other organs.

### ABCD system

Some doctors use this older and more traditional cancer staging system, in which A and B represent cancer that's confined to the prostate gland, and C and D indicate cancer that has spread to other parts of the body.

Like the TNM system, each capital letter in the ABCD system is followed by a subcategory that represents details in the staging. Because the ABCD system has fewer categories, it's less precise.

## Survival statistics

Thanks to advances in both detection and treatment, survival rates for prostate cancer have improved considerably during the past two decades. For example, in 1981 the five-year survival rate for all men with prostate cancer was 74 percent. That survival rate had risen to 97 percent by 1998 with professionals forecasting a continuing decline in mortality. Today, about 79 percent of all men with prostate cancer live at least 10 years, and 57 percent live 15 years or more. Black men continue to have lower survival rates than do white men (see charts on the right).

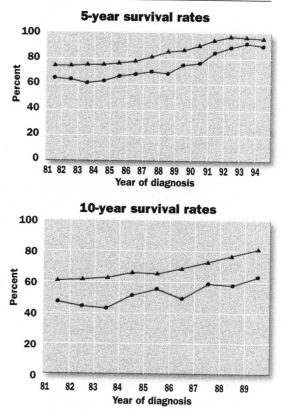

The top line of each graph (▲) shows survival rates for whites. The bottom line (●) shows rates for blacks.

Adapted from: National Cancer Institute's Surveillance, Epidemiology and End Results (SEER) program

It's hoped that survival figures will continue to improve if more men have regular digital rectal examinations and PSA tests to identify cancer during early stages, when it can be cured. For cancer that's diagnosed early and confined to the prostate, the survival rate is almost 100 percent.

## Answers to your questions

*What are tumor markers?*
These are substances made from cancerous cells found in the blood. When they exist in elevated levels, they may indicate the presence of cancer. During treatment and follow-up visits, your blood may

be routinely checked for elevated tumor markers. PSA is a tumor marker for prostate cancer.

*Is a biopsy the only way I can be sure I have prostate cancer?*
Yes. Other tests, such as a digital rectal examination or PSA test, can suggest a strong possibility of prostate cancer. But a biopsy is the only way to be certain.

*Can a biopsy be wrong?*
When tissue samples are taken from the gland, it's possible to miss the cancer. This is called a sampling error. A biopsy result that comes back normal isn't a guarantee that you don't have cancer. Sampling errors, however, are uncommon.

*Can a biopsy loosen cancer cells, allowing them to spread?*
No evidence suggests that this can happen. Cancer cells not removed in the biopsy stay within the tumor where they have been growing.

*Why do I need to stop taking aspirin before a biopsy?*
Aspirin and some other pain medications thin your blood and can increase your risk of bleeding. Discontinuing these medications for a short period before and after a prostate biopsy will reduce your chances of serious bleeding from the procedure. The same is true for prescription blood thinners, taken to reduce clotting, such as warfarin (Coumadin).

*Is it possible for a biopsy to cause permanent impotence?*
No. Impotence that follows a biopsy is probably due to stress that often accompanies cancer diagnosis and treatment. In some cases it may result from temporary inflammation.

*Can I pass cancer on to my wife during sexual intercourse?*
No. Cancer cells won't escape from your body through intercourse. Even if they could, they wouldn't be able to grow inside another person because they're genetically coded for your body.

## Chapter 7

# What are your options?

F inding out you have cancer can lead to panic. You may feel as if you need to make an instant decision and begin your treatment right away. However, because prostate cancer is often a slow-growing cancer, there's generally no need to rush.

Give yourself time to gather some information and consider your treatment options. You may want to visit a patient education library, if your local hospital or medical center has one. Or you can stop at your local library or check out well-respected sources on the Internet, such as the American Cancer Society, American Urological Association and the National Comprehensive Cancer Network. While you're learning about your condition, write down questions you want to ask your doctor before the two of you decide on a treatment plan.

You may also find it helpful to take a family member or friend with you to your next appointment. He or she can remind you of important questions you want to ask. That person can also listen and help you recall the discussion afterward, including important points made.

Often, there's more than one way to treat prostate cancer. Some men may benefit from a combination of two or more treatment options, such as surgery followed by radiation. Which treatment you and your doctor choose will depend on several factors, such as how fast the cancer is growing, how much it has spread, your age and overall health, as well as the benefits and potential side effects.

## Letting the cancer alone

Because blood tests can now help detect prostate cancer at a very early stage, more men have more options earlier in the process. One option is to forgo treatment and monitor for signs and symptoms of progression. This approach goes by several names, including *watchful waiting, observation* or *expectant therapy.* You do nothing except keep a close watch on the cancer with regular blood tests and digital rectal examinations, performed about every six months. You may also need to have occasional biopsies.

If you're fairly young and healthy, in your 50s or 60s, your doctor may not recommend this approach. Because of your age, the cancer has many years to grow, and even a small, slow-growing cancer might eventually reach the point when it needs treatment. The cancer cells could also become aggressive and spread so much that a cure becomes difficult or impossible.

However, if you're in your 70s or older and the cancer is small and slow-growing, watchful waiting might be an option. A study by Swedish researchers published in 2002 followed about 700 men with prostate cancer whose average age was 65. It found that those who selected surgery were less likely to have cancer that spread beyond the prostate and less likely to die of the disease than were men who chose watchful waiting. However, after six years, the overall survival rates for the two groups were similar. That's because men in the surgery group died from unrelated causes at a slightly higher rate than did men in the watchful waiting group.

With careful monitoring, you and your doctor can act quickly if the cancer does become aggressive, and treatment becomes necessary to stop or slow its growth.

### Are you a candidate for watchful waiting?
You may be a candidate for watchful waiting if:
- You're age 70 or older with a small cancer (Gleason score of less than 6)
- The cancer is confined to the prostate and you want time to think about your options

- You're unable to withstand the side effects of treatment for age or health reasons
- Your life expectancy is less than 10 years, because of another condition

## What are the benefits?

- You avoid the risks, such as impotence or incontinence, associated with other treatments,.
- Watchful waiting buys you time to consider treatment options. It can take several years for a tiny tumor to double in size, and you can use this time to your benefit.
- It's the least expensive option, requiring only occasional exams and tests.

## What are the disadvantages?

- The cancer can grow while you wait. Although rare, a slow-growing cancer may turn into a faster-growing cancer. For example, in a study published in 2001, about 13 percent of men showed a significant change in grade of Gleason scores from 6 or less to 7 or greater during a period of about two years. In such cases, the cancer may require more extensive treatment that results in greater side effects than if it had been treated earlier.
- You may become what's been called walking worried, always anxious about your cancer and preoccupied with your tests and condition. Although more aggressive treatment has risks, it may reduce the fear that you're gambling with your life.

## Removing the prostate gland

Surgical removal of the prostate gland is a direct and effective means of treating many cases of prostate cancer. This type of surgery is called radical prostatectomy.

The majority of men in their 40s and 50s, and many in their 60s, choose radical prostatectomy. More men in their 70s prefer radiation therapy to surgery, and men in their 80s tend to choose no therapy.

New procedures and instruments developed during the past two decades have changed this surgery considerably. Surgeons now use

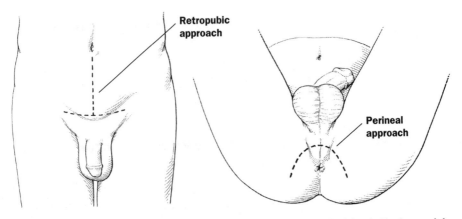

With retropubic surgery, the prostate gland is removed through an incision in the lower abdomen. Perineal surgery involves removing the gland through an incision between the anus and the scrotal sac.

special techniques to remove the prostate, while sparing muscles and attached nerve bundles that control urination and sexual function. Improvements in techniques that control bleeding have resulted in a dramatic reduction in blood loss and in the need for transfusion.

### Retropubic prostatectomy

Retropubic surgery is the most common of two methods for removing the prostate. In this procedure, the gland is taken out through an incision in the lower abdomen that typically runs from just below the navel to an inch above the penis (see illustration).

It's the most common form of prostate removal for two reasons. The surgeon can use the same incision to remove surrounding lymph nodes, which are tested to determine whether the cancer has spread beyond the prostate. In addition, the procedure gives the surgeon better access to the prostate, making it easier to save the nerve bundles that control erection.

The night before surgery you'll likely be given an enema or laxatives to clear your rectum of any fecal matter. This reduces the chance of infection if the rectal wall is punctured during surgery, an uncommon but possible risk.

You may choose general anesthesia during the surgery, or you may chose to remain awake and have spinal (epidural) anesthesia, which numbs only the lower half of your body. General anesthesia is more common.

After the incision, the surgeon may remove lymph nodes near your prostate and send samples to a pathologist. Enlarged or suspect lymph nodes can be evaluated by frozen-section techniques to determine if cancer is present. Results are often known within 15 to 30 minutes. If cancer is found, your surgeon may close the incision without removing the gland or may proceed with the surgery. The decision to proceed in light of positive lymph nodes depends on the number of lymph nodes involved, your age and associated symptoms. The fewer nodes that contain cancer, the younger your age and the fewer symptoms you have, the more likely your doctor will be to continue with surgery.

Removal of the prostate requires detaching it from the bottom of the bladder. The urethra is also severed below the prostate gland (see image below), but above the external (urethral) sphincter that helps to control urine flow. The vasa deferentia, which carry sperm from the testicles to the urethra, enter the urinary channel through the back of the prostate and also must be cut in order to remove the prostate. The seminal vesicles are attached to the prostate and are a potential site for the spread of prostate cancer. These vesicles are removed along with the prostate gland. The surgeon will then re-attach your urethra to your bladder below the site of the now-removed prostate. This re-connection allows you to urinate normally, although it may take several days to a few weeks — or in some cases months — for your body to heal enough for you to regain bladder control.

Depending on where the cancer is, your surgeon will try to save the nerve bundles attached to each side of the prostate. These nerves control your ability to have an erection. Surgeons can often spare one or both of these bundles.

Men in their 40s and 50s who have this nerve-sparing

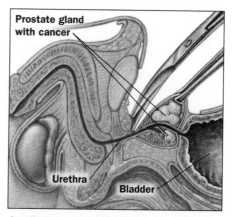

A radical prostatectomy involves removing the prostate gland (shown here with cancerous tissue) and seminal vesicles. The urethra, which is cut to allow removal of the prostate, is reattached just below the bladder.

surgery are more likely to retain their ability to have an erection than are older men. For some older men — especially those not sexually active — the spared nerves don't survive the shock of surgery. On average, half the men who are sexually active before surgery experience impotence or diminished sexual functioning after surgery.

If even one nerve bundle is spared, it's still possible to have erections. If neither nerve bundle can be spared, it's unlikely that you'll have normal erections without treatment. Even if your ability to have erections is lost, you can still have a normal sex drive (libido), your sensation is unchanged, and you can still have orgasms (sexual climax). Devices and medications that can help you achieve an erection if you can no longer do so naturally are discussed in Chapter 9.

Regardless of whether or not your ability to have erections is preserved after surgery, or is restored with treatment, no fluid

## Following surgery

Before you leave the hospital, you'll receive instructions from your doctor about caring for yourself after your surgery. The following may be part of your recovery routine.

A urinary catheter will be in place to promote healing of the junction where your ureter was reattached to your bladder. You'll receive instructions on catheter care. Follow the instructions carefully. They are designed to help prevent infection and blockage of urine.

Adequate consumption of fluids is especially important in the weeks while the catheter is in place. This will help keep urine flowing freely and reduce chance of a blockage.

A medication chart may also be useful. List the medications you're taking daily on a sheet of paper. Include check-off spaces for dosages and times (a.m., p.m. or both).

Try to avoid constipation during the healing period. Eat plenty of fruits and vegetables and avoid red meat and pork for a couple of months. It's important not to have enemas or rectal examinations for a few months following surgery.

Don't become a couch potato during your recovery. Staying

(ejaculate) will be produced with an orgasm. That's because the structures that make and transport semen and sperm — the prostate, seminal vesicles and vasa deferentia — have either been removed or disconnected. The fact that you have dry orgasms has no effect on sensation, but it does mean that you won't be able to father children without medical help.

After surgery, recovery in the hospital for one to three days, and three to five weeks at home, is typical. You'll also need to use a catheter for about two to three weeks to give your urinary tract time to heal.

### Perineal prostatectomy

With this form of surgery, an incision is made between the anus and the scrotal sac, which holds the testicles. There's generally less bleeding with perineal surgery, and heavier men generally recover sooner with this surgery than they do with retropubic prostatectomy. Unfortunately, this approach makes it much more difficult — and

active is important, and walking is an excellent form of exercise. Movement helps prevent the development of blood clots in your legs. See your doctor if you develop redness or tenderness in the area of a leg vein. Clots can become life-threatening.

When your catheter is removed, you may experience leakage of urine. That's because it takes time to resolve the swelling in the muscles that help keep you dry and for those muscles to regain their strength. You may need diapers for a few days or more, and an absorbent pad after that. Muscle strengthening exercises may be helpful. Take the time and effort to perform these simple exercises daily (see "Strengthening your pelvic floor muscles" on page 109). They can help reduce or eliminate your incontinence, but be patient. This may take a year or more. A sense of humor about wearing diapers temporarily will also serve you well.

Incontinence over time can cause a rash near the tip of your penis. This is a yeast infection called balanitis. Your doctor can prescribe an antifungal cream. Wash your penis with soap and water daily and dry thoroughly before applying the cream, which clears up the infection and can help prevent a recurrence.

sometimes impossible — for your surgeon to locate and save the nerve bundles attached to the prostate. In addition, the surgeon isn't able to reach nearby lymph nodes. That's why this surgery is less commonly used.

### Are you a candidate for surgery?
You may be a candidate for surgery if:
- Your cancer is confined to the prostate gland
- You're healthy enough to withstand surgery
- Your expected life span is greater than the life span the cancer would allow

### What are the benefits?
For cancer that's confined to the prostate gland, surgery is a very effective treatment. It can cure your disease.

### What are the disadvantages?
- All major surgery carries some risk of death. For radical prostatectomy, that risk is quite low. One large study of more than 100,000 men showed the 30-day mortality rate due to complications after surgery was less than 0.5 percent for men ages 65 to 69 and close to 1 percent for men age 75 and older.
- You may become impotent. This depends a lot on your age. A study published in 1999 involving more than 1,800 men who had radical retropubic prostatectomies with nerve-sparing found that 80 percent under age 60 regained potency, compared with 60 percent of men in their 60s and 47 percent of those in their 70s. The American Cancer Society says that some cancer centers in the United States report potency rates of 70 percent to 75 percent for men under 60 who have nerve-sparing surgery, and rates of 20 percent to 30 percent in men over 70 who have the same surgery. The skill of your surgeon and the quality of your erections before surgery also can affect the outcome. If you had trouble achieving or maintaining an erection before surgery, the chances are greater that you'll be impotent after surgery.
- You may experience incontinence — at least temporarily. After the catheter is removed, nearly all men have some bladder-

control problems for at least a few days. You could have problems for weeks, or even months. If so, medications and treatment can help improve bladder control. About 90 percent of men eventually regain complete control where continence is defined as no regular use of pads or no leakage during moderate exercise. About 5 percent to 10 percent of men experience stress incontinence, meaning they can't hold their urine flow when pressure is placed on the bladder, as happens when they sneeze, cough, laugh or lift.

- Recovery can take one to two months or longer.
- There's a small risk of damage to your lower intestine or rectum. More surgery may be necessary to repair the damage.

## Destroying the cancer with radiation

Radiation treatment uses high-powered X-rays or other radiation to kill cancer cells. Radiation is effective in treating cancer because it interferes with cancer cells' ability to reproduce. Cancer cells are also generally more susceptible to radiation's harmful effects than are normal cells. Radiation is used to treat many different types of cancer and has been used to treat prostate cancer for decades.

Radiation is also used to treat cancer that has spread outside the prostate. It can destroy cancerous cells, shrink tumors and relieve painful symptoms.

### External beam therapy

Radiation is most commonly delivered by a large machine — called a linear accelerator — that produces a concentrated beam that's focused on the prostate gland. Because radiation can damage healthy tissue in the same area of the prostate — including the bladder and rectum — precise positioning and aiming are used to reduce side effects.

A first step in radiation therapy is to map the areas in your body to receive radiation. Three-dimensional scans show the location of the prostate and surrounding organs. Computer imaging software allows a radiation therapist to rotate the picture in any direction to find the best angles to fire the beams.

Treatments are generally given five days a week for about six to eight weeks. Each treatment takes about 15 minutes. However, much of this is preparation time. The actual length of time you receive radiation may be only a few minutes. To make sure the beams are always precisely on the mark, you'll have a body supporter that will hold you in the same position for each treatment. You'll also be asked to arrive with a full bladder, which will help hold your prostate in the same position during each treatment. Ink marks on your skin will help the radiation therapist hit the same targets each time. Custom-designed shields cover nearby areas such as your intestines, anus, rectal wall and urethra, protecting them from scattered rays.

In addition, a relatively new procedure uses small metallic markers to more precisely determine the position of the prostate before each treatment. These markers are inserted into the prostate using a method similar to that used to biopsy prostate tissue. Once implanted, imaging equipment built into the X-ray machine determines the best position of the beam for maximum effect and least damage to surrounding tissue. Another method of localizing external beam therapy uses ultrasound to scan the prostate from a small transducer placed on the lower abdomen.

During the radiation treatments, you'll lie on a table while the linear accelerator moves above you, targeting the cancer with radiation.

Another type of external beam therapy uses protons instead of X-rays to kill the cancer. Protons are parts of atoms that cause little damage to surrounding tissue but effectively destroy cells at the end of the beam. The protons travel through noncancerous tissue and come to rest in the targeted area, where they deposit their radiation dose. This allows your therapist to deliver stronger doses of beam radiation. This form of radiation therapy is under study at a few medical centers.

External beam therapy is also used after surgery to treat the area around where the prostate used to be — the prostate bed. This may be done when microscopic examination of prostate tissue indicates that small amounts of cancer cells may have been left behind after surgery. Such treatment is to reduce the chance that the cancer will grow back. In these circumstances, radiation treatments are usually given no sooner than two to three months after surgery and they last from six to seven weeks — a somewhat shorter time than when radiation therapy is performed as the primary treatment. Radiation may also be given if your prostate-specific antigen level starts to rise some months or years after surgery.

### Radioactive seed implants

Another method of delivering radiation to cancer cells within the prostate is called brachytherapy (brak-e-THER-uh-pe). It uses ultrasound-guided needles to inject rice-sized radioactive seeds, or pellets, into your prostate (see illustration). These seeds deliver double the dose of radiation of external beams. Brachytherapy may be used alone or in combination with external beam therapy or hormone therapy.

The procedure is done on an outpatient basis, with either general anesthesia or spinal (epidural) anesthesia, which numbs the lower portion of your body.

Between 70 and 150 seeds are inserted in and around your prostate through hollow needles that pass through the skin of your perineum, the area between your scrotum and anus. The number of seeds inserted depends on the size of your prostate. The seed-implant procedure is generally more easily performed on small or moderate-sized prostates.

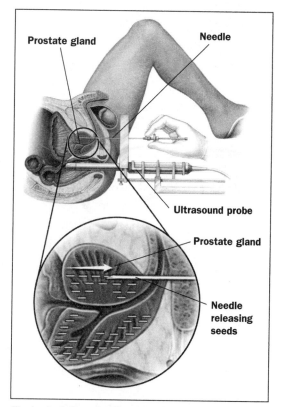

The implantation of radioactive seeds, or pellets, to treat prostate cancer (brachytherapy) usually takes about two hours. An ultrasound probe is placed in the rectum to help guide placement of the seeds. The seeds, which emit radiation that damages or kills cancer cells, usually remain in place permanently.

Depending on the grade of your cancer, one of several radioactive substances — called isotopes — will be used in the brachtherapy seeds. The most commonly used low-energy isotopes are iodine 125 and palladium (puh-LA-de-um) 103. The seeds remain in the prostate permanently, even after they stop emitting radiation. Other seeds that contain a more potent substance, called iridium (ih-RID-e-um), are left in temporarily in a treatment known as high-dose-rate (HDR) afterloading brachytherapy. HDR afterloading brachytherapy is considered temporary because the seeds are eventually removed. Permanent-seed brachytherapy is more common because HDR treatments are usually given in combination with four to five weeks of external beam therapy, which makes HDR less convenient for the patient.

An ultrasound probe inserted into your rectum guides the doctor in placing the seeds in and around your prostate. A template attached to the outside of the probe and held up against your perineum guides and steadies the needles loaded with seeds.

Iodine and palladium seeds generally emit radiation only a few millimeters beyond where they're implanted. Although this type of radiation isn't thought to escape your prostate area, doctors recommend that for the first couple of months after implantation you minimize prolonged close (less than 2 feet) contact with small children and pregnant women, who are especially sensitive to radiation. Within a year, all radiation inside the pellets is generally exhausted.

Studies have shown that brachytherapy has controlled or halted cancer growth for five years in 90 percent of men and for 10 years in 70 percent to 85 percent of men.

Radioactive seed implants generally produce side effects that are similar to those from external beam therapy. They may cause more temporary side effects involving urination — including increased frequency and burning — than does external beam therapy.

### Are you a candidate for radiation?
You may be a candidate for radiation therapy if:
- Your cancer can't be cured by surgery because it has spread outside the prostate
- You don't want surgery

- You expect to live longer than your cancer would allow you to live

## What are the benefits?

- Radiation treatment is an effective treatment. It can cure your disease.
- The procedure is generally done on an outpatient basis. With brachytherapy, you may need to spend one night in the hospital.
- External beam therapy is a noninvasive treatment that doesn't require anesthesia.
- Radiation doesn't involve the rigors and recovery associated with surgery.

## What are the disadvantages?

- Radiation can affect your sexual function. Over time, it can damage the nerves that control erections and the arteries that carry blood to your penis. Most men don't have problems with erections or intercourse in the early months after radiation therapy. But eventually many experience some complications.

## 10 questions to ask your doctor

To help determine the best form of treatment for you, ask your doctor these questions:

1. What options are available?
2. How fast will the cancer grow if left untreated?
3. Do you think the cancer can be cured with treatment? If so, what are the chances?
4. Which treatment would you recommend, and why?
5. How many times have you performed this procedure?
6. How soon before we know if the treatment has worked?
7. What are the risks of lasting side effects, such as impotence or incontinence?
8. How soon is it possible to return to work?
9. Will any activities have to be restricted?
10. If the treatment doesn't work, are there other options?

A summary of 11 studies published between 1999 and 2001 of men treated with external beam therapy found that between 41 percent and 85 percent experienced at least some degree of erectile dysfunction (ED). A man's age and the amount of radiation he received affected his chances of experiencing ED after treatment. The same summary showed the rate of ED after brachytherapy was somewhat lower. It ranged between 30 percent and 53 percent. Generally, the younger you are, the better your chance of retaining the ability to have normal sexual function after treatment.

- Some men have bowel problems from external beam therapy, including increased frequency of bowel movements, rectal bleeding, a burning feeling around the anus, and a sense that you need to have a bowel movement. The signs and symptoms generally subside when the treatments are over. But for about 3 percent of men, the signs and symptoms may persist for a year or may require treatment.

- External beam therapy produces urinary problems in approximately one in three men. Some studies have shown that less than 1 percent of men treated with brachytherapy develop long-term urinary incontinence. The most common complaints are constantly feeling as if you have to urinate and a burning sensation while urinating. Blood in your urine or urine leakage are less common. Less than 1 percent need surgery to correct a problem.

## Freezing the cancer cells

Another way to kill prostate cancer is to freeze prostate tissue. Doctors use a similar approach to kill warts, dipping a swab into a tank of supercooled liquid nitrogen, then swabbing the wart, which eventually dies and falls off. Prostate tissue dies in the same way and is absorbed and then eliminated by your body.

Called cryotherapy, or cryoablation, the procedure involves inserting five to seven thin metal rods, each about 6 inches long, through the perineum and into the prostate. An ultrasound probe in the rectum helps your doctor position the rods. Once the rod tips are in place, liquid nitrogen is released into the rods, where it circulates and plunges the temperature to about minus 374 F. As the tissue freezes, the formation and expansion of ice crystals within the cancerous cells cause them to rupture and die. To keep the urethra from freezing along with your prostate, a catheter is placed inside the urethra and filled with a warming solution.

The entire procedure takes about two hours, with most of the time used to carefully position the rods and about 30 minutes to freeze the prostate.

You can expect to stay in the hospital one to two days. You'll probably be able to return to your normal activities in a couple of weeks. However, it will take your body about nine months to a year to shed the dead cells. The procedure may have to be repeated.

### Are you a candidate for cryotherapy?

You may be a candidate for cryotherapy if:

- Your cancer is confined to the prostate
- You're not healthy enough to withstand surgery
- You don't want surgery or radiation therapy

### What are the advantages?

- Cryotherapy has been shown to control cancer confined to the prostate in 60 percent to 75 percent of men five years after treatment.
- The procedure requires only one or two days in the hospital and can sometimes be done on an outpatient basis.
- There's very little blood loss.
- Recovery time is short, just one or two weeks.

### What are the disadvantages?

- The procedure is fairly new and not widely used.
- Cryotherapy doesn't always kill all of the cancer cells on the first try. It may have to be repeated.
- You have an 80-percent to 90-percent chance of developing impotence because nerve bundles that control erections can freeze and die.
- You may have trouble urinating for several weeks. Freezing swells the prostate temporarily, which squeezes the urethra.

- You'll have temporary soreness where the rods were inserted.
- Although the short-term results look encouraging, long-term survival rates appear lower than do those with surgery or radiation therapy.

## Answers to your questions

*Is surgery more difficult in some men?*
Radical prostatectomy can be more challenging in men who are obese or who have an especially deep or narrow pelvis. A very large prostate also can be more challenging to remove. However, a skilled surgeon should be able to overcome these obstacles.

*Isn't radiation harmful?*
Radiation can be harmful to normal tissue if it's given in excess. That's why the amount you receive during radiation therapy is precisely calculated and controlled to minimize damage to healthy cells.

*Can the radioactive seeds work their way out of the prostate gland?*
Occasionally some seeds can get into the urethra and be excreted in your urine. This generally doesn't cause problems. Seeds may also infrequently become dislodged from the prostate and travel through the bloodstream to other parts of the body, typically the chest and lungs. The number of seeds that may migrate is very small — less than 1 percent — and no side effects have been reported. A new type of seed that's built into an absorbable strand is designed to reduce the chance that seeds will migrate.

*Should I get a second opinion before making a decision?*
If you feel confident in your doctor and comfortable with your treatment plan, a second opinion may not be necessary. However, if you have concerns about your diagnosis, you don't feel confident in your doctor, or you don't feel comfortable with the proposed treatment, then you may want another opinion. If you're considering all treatment options, reviewing these options with different specialists is recommended.

## Chapter 8

# When the cancer is advanced

For cancer that has spread outside the prostate gland, treating the disease becomes more difficult. However, certain treatments can help slow its growth and even shrink the tumors. This means an opportunity for you to live longer and enjoy a better quality of life, even though you may have advanced cancer.

## Controlling the cancer with hormones

Many prostate cancers feed off androgens — from the Greek words *andros* (man) and *gennan* (to produce). These male sex hormones produce male characteristics. Testosterone, the main male sex hormone, is responsible for the normal development of sex organs and other male features, such as facial hair and large muscles.

When you have prostate cancer, the circulation of male sex hormones throughout your body and around the cancer makes the cancer grow faster. The most common way to treat advanced prostate cancer is to drastically reduce or cut off the supply of these hormones to the cancer. Hormone therapy — sometimes called androgen deprivation therapy — uses drugs or testicular removal to do one or two things, sometimes both. It can:

- Stop production of most, but not all, male sex hormones.
- Block remaining hormones from getting into cancer cells.

Hormone therapy is so effective at shrinking tumors that it's being used in some early-stage prostate cancers, too, in combination with surgery and radiation therapy. The hormones shrink large tumors so that radiation can destroy them more easily. And after radiation, the drugs can help kill stray cells left behind at the tumor site.

A study published in 2002 found that 74 percent of men who had both external beam therapy and hormone therapy were disease-free after five years, compared with 40 percent of men who received only radiation. Overall survival was 78 percent of men who had both treatments, compared with 62 percent of men who received radiation alone.

There are four different types of hormone therapy.

### Drugs that decrease testosterone production

More than 90 percent of testosterone is produced by the testicles. One hormone treatment sets up a chemical blockade, preventing the testicles from receiving messages to make testosterone. These messages initially come from the hypothalamus, an area of your brain that secretes chemicals to control many body functions. One of these chemicals is luteinizing hormone-releasing hormone (LH-RH). It alerts the pituitary gland, located just below your brain, to release luteinizing hormone (LH), the chemical that signals your testicles to make testosterone.

Several medications known as LH-RH agonists can interrupt this message pathway. The medications are synthetic hormones similar to your brain's natural LH-RH. But instead of turning on the chemical switch that activates LH, they turn it off. Your testicles never get the message to produce testosterone.

Two of the more common LH-RH blockers are leuprolide (Lupron, Viadur) and goserelin (Zoladex). These are given periodically by injection.

### Drugs that block hormone use

Not all testosterone is produced in the testicles. Around 5 percent to 10 percent comes from the adrenal glands, located on top of each of your kidneys. Medications known as antiandrogens keep this testosterone away from the cancer cells.

The drugs compete with testosterone for entrance into the cancer cells, eventually crowding out the testosterone. Three drugs, which come in tablet form, are most frequently used. They are flutamide (Eulexin, generics), bicalutamide (Casodex) and nilutamide (Nilandron). Depending on the brand of drug you're prescribed, you take the medication one to three times a day.

Anti-androgen therapy is often used in combination with LH-RH drugs, resulting in little or no testosterone getting to the cancer cells. Doctors refer to the combination as total androgen blockade.

## Intermittent drug use

Depriving prostate cancer of testosterone usually doesn't kill the cancer. Within one to three years, the cancer often becomes resistant and begins to thrive without testosterone. Once this happens, options to stop the cancer are limited.

Some researchers suspect that continuous use of hormone medications may be the reason the cancer adapts. These researchers believe that taking breaks from the medication might keep the cancer from adjusting to the testosterone loss, or at least slow the process. The long-term benefits of intermittent drug therapy have yet to be proven. Results of clinical studies may be known in about three years.

Exactly how prostate cancer cells become resistant is unclear. There are many different kinds of prostate cancer cells. Two broad categories are hormone-sensitive cancer cells and hormone-insensitive cancer cells. When you get prostate cancer, you probably have some of both. The more hormone-sensitive cells you have, the better you'll respond to hormone treatment. The fewer you have, the less you'll respond. In time, the hormone-sensitive cells die, and the hormone-insensitive cells increase.

With intermittent therapy, you stop taking hormone drugs after your prostate-specific antigen (PSA) drops to a low level and remains steady. You resume the drugs when your PSA level rises again, generally above 10 nanograms per milliliter. During the drug-free periods, which can last a year or more, you may not be bothered by side effects of the medications, which may include decreased sex drive, impotence and breast enlargement (gynecomastia).

### Are you a candidate for hormone drug therapy?
If your cancer has spread beyond the prostate gland, you may benefit from hormone therapy.

### What are the benefits?
- Hormone drug therapy can temporarily slow the growth of prostate cancer and shrink existing tumors, reducing your symptoms and allowing you to live longer.
- It's approximately 80-percent effective on average for one to three years.
- It may be stopped, sometimes allowing the return of normal hormone production.

### What are the disadvantages?
- Hormone drug therapy lowers or eliminates the sex drive in most men.
- It often causes impotence.
- It can cause hot flashes, similar to those women often experience during menopause.
- It may cause your breasts to slightly enlarge and become sore. Low doses of radiation treatment can prevent this.
- It produces weight gain, often 10 to 15 pounds.
- It reduces your muscle and bone mass, making you more prone to broken bones (osteoporosis).
- Some drugs cause nausea, diarrhea and fatigue.
- In rare cases it can lead to liver damage.
- Most cancers become resistant to the medication on average in one to three years.
- Some medications can cost hundreds of dollars a month and may not be covered by insurance.

With current hormone drug therapy, about 50 percent of men whose cancer has spread to other pelvic organs, such as the bladder and the rectum, live for five years. About 40 percent live for 10 years. If the cancer has spread to bone, time is often shortened. In such cases, about 50 percent of men live two years and approximately 30 percent live five years.

### Testicular surgery

Surgically removing the testicles to prevent testosterone production was once the standard treatment for advanced prostate cancer. It's still done, but hormone-blocking drugs have reduced the use of testicular surgery by providing what amounts to chemical castration.

*Bilateral orchiectomy* (or-ke-EK-tuh-me) is the medical term for testicle removal. *Orchi* is from the Greek word *orchis* meaning "testicle," and *ectomy* means "removal." *Bilateral* refers to the fact that both testicles are removed. Orchiectomy is as effective as hormone drug therapy in limiting the production of testosterone.

The procedure is often performed on an outpatient basis using a local anesthetic. The doctor will make a small incision at the center of your scrotum, the pouch that holds your testicles. Each testicle is clipped from the attached spermatic cord and removed. Most of the cord is left for a natural appearance. Some men have an artificial testicular implant placed into the scrotum during the surgery, to maintain a more normal appearance.

### Are you a candidate for orchiectomy?

You may benefit from an orchiectomy if:

- You can't tolerate hormone drug therapy for health reasons unrelated to your prostate cancer.
- You aren't able to take daily medication as prescribed, or regularly visit the doctor's office for hormone injections.

### What are the benefits?

- Orchiectomy is performed on an outpatient basis.
- The risk of complications is low.
- It's less expensive than hormone medications.
- Its effects are almost immediate. Within a few hours, the only testosterone left is the small amount coming from your adrenal glands.
- The side effects may be less intense than with medications.

### What are the disadvantages?

- As with hormone medications, orchiectomy reduces or eliminates the sex drive in most men.

- Orchiectomy leaves most men impotent.
- Some men experience breast enlargement or soreness.
- Approximately half the men experience hot flashes.
- You may feel less masculine and become depressed, like the feelings a woman may have after breast removal or a hysterectomy.
- It can lead to osteoporosis, a disorder that weakens your bones and increases your risk of fractures.
- Though your cancer will probably go into remission for one to three years, it will almost certainly return, because the cancer cells adapt to the absence of hormones.

After bilateral orchiectomy for metastatic prostate cancer, about 50 percent of men live three more years. About 25 percent live five years or more. Men with cancer confined to the pelvic area generally live longer — 50 percent to 60 percent live five years, and 40 percent live 10 years or more.

## Using chemotherapy

Chemotherapy is part of first-line treatment for some cancers. In treating prostate cancer, chemotherapy is more often used in situations when the cancer has continued to grow and spread despite other forms of treatment, including hormonal therapy.

As the name suggests, chemotherapy uses chemicals — specifically, anti-cancer drugs — to destroy cancer cells. These drugs may be given intravenously, by injection, or in pill form. Unfortunately, chemotherapy may have unpleasant side effects because anti-cancer drugs are toxic to healthy cells as well as cancer cells. Common side effects may include hair loss, nausea, vomiting, fatigue, changes in bowel function and lowered resistance to infection. The severity of side effects varies from person to person. In some, the side effects may be mild, while in others they're more pronounced.

Chemotherapy may sometimes relieve the symptoms of advanced prostate cancer, such as pain resulting from the cancer. However, to date chemotherapy hasn't been shown to extend life in men with advanced prostate cancer.

### Are you a candidate for chemotherapy?

Your doctor may recommend chemotherapy if hormonal therapy is no longer working and your general medical condition is stable enough to try this treatment.

### What are the benefits?

Chemotherapy may relieve pain and other symptoms related to your prostate cancer. The medications may slow the growth of prostate cancer in some men.

### What are the disadvantages?

Chemotherapy hasn't worked as well in treating prostate cancer as it has for some other forms of cancer. In addition, some side effects may lead to discomfort while others may be more serious, such as a compromised immune system that can lower your ability to fight infection.

## Trying an experimental procedure

If traditional treatments are unable to control the cancer, your doctor may suggest that you consider participating in a clinical trial. Some trials involve traditional chemotherapy treatments, but in new variations or combinations.

Other trials may involve experimental treatments with new drugs. These treatments may range from ones that have been used in several people and the side effects to which are already known, while other treatments may be very new and cause unexpected side effects.

### Gene and immunotherapy

Your immune system is capable of attacking cancerous cells, but it often can't differentiate them from normal cells. Researchers are studying ways of genetically altering prostate cancer cells in the laboratory to make them more recognizable as foreign invaders. The altered cells would then be injected back into your body to help your immune system better recognize and destroy all prostate cancer cells.

Another approach, still in the theory stage, would involve injecting into the body genes modified to attack only prostate cancer cells. These modified genes would be coded to switch on only when they came into contact with prostate cancer cells, limiting damage to healthy cells.

### Experimental chemotherapy

Another area of research is focused on how prostate cancer cells can be made more sensitive — and vulnerable — to chemotherapy. This strategy has had some success in treating some forms of breast cancer with a drug called trastuzumab (Herceptin). Trastuzumab blocks the product of a gene abnormality in breast cancer.

To find out more about clinical studies taking place in these areas, ask your doctor or contact a cancer organization, such as the National Cancer Institute (see "Additional resources" on page 173).

## Strategies for relieving pain

Early-stage prostate cancer typically isn't painful. However, once the cancer spreads beyond the gland to nearby bone, it may produce intense pain. This pain isn't something you need to live with. There are many effective methods for relieving the difficult pain of cancer.

### Treating local pain

If you experience pain in a specific area of your body, such as your lower back, you have these options for treating it:

**External radiation.** External beam therapy is frequently used to treat painful sites where prostate cancer has spread. In such cases, this treatment is usually effective between 50 percent and 80 percent of the time in completely or partially relieving symptoms.

**Strontium and samarium.** Pain from advanced cancer often comes from cancer that has spread to the bones. The radioactive elements strontium and samarium are effective in relieving this kind of pain. After you receive an injection of either strontium or samarium, the radioactive element is carried to your bones where it's absorbed. Cancerous bones absorb more of the radioactive substance than do healthy bones. This helps concentrate most of the drug at the source of your pain. Most men feel better after a single injection.

Effects from these radioactive drugs can last several weeks or months. In some circumstances, they may last up to a year. If you find these injections helpful, you may receive more than one, but usually no more frequently than once every two months. Depending on the dose given and the substance used, your urine may be radioactive for the first few days after the injection and you must dispose of it in a hazardous waste container.

As a result of this treatment, your white blood cell and blood platelet counts may decrease, putting you at increased risk of a serious infection. Because of this, periodic testing to monitor your blood counts will likely be done.

**External beam radiation and strontium or samarium.** Often, an effective way to relieve localized bone pain is to combine these treatments.

**Nerve stimulators.** Although not widely used for pain associated with prostate cancer, transcutaneous electrical nerve stimulation (TENS) offers relief for some men. Small electrodes are attached to your skin near the pain site. These electrodes are then wired to a small battery-powered unit you can clip onto your belt. Gentle electrical pulses travel to the electrodes and divert your pain-sensing nerves.

**Nerve blocks.** Specialists in anesthesiology can inject numbing analgesics into nerves at the site of your pain. This works especially well if your pain is in a specific area where nerves can be identified and targeted.

### Treating general pain

If you experience pain related to your cancer, try to rate it on a scale of 1 to 10, with 1 being no pain and 10 being the worst pain imaginable (see graph on page 102). This will help establish the best course of treatment.

**Medications.** If your pain is mild and no more bothersome than a headache, an over-the-counter pain reliever may be all you need. If your pain is more intense, you may need a stronger prescription medication. Discuss this with your doctor.

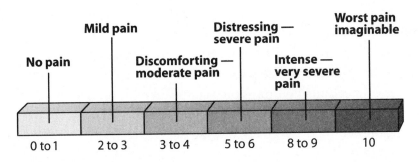

Use this scale as a guide to determine your level of pain.

Opioids (narcotics) are commonly taken to relieve cancer pain. Some opioids are natural compounds derived from opium. Others are synthetic drugs that work in a similar manner. Opioids include:

- Codeine
- Fentanyl (Duragesic)
- Hydrocodone (Lorcet, Lortab)
- Hydromorphone (Dilaudid)
- Levorphanol (Levo-Dromoran)
- Meperidine (Demerol)
- Methadone (Dolophine)
- Morphine (MS Contin, Oramorph SR, others)
- Oxycodone (OxyContin)
- Oxymorphone (Numorphan)
- Propoxyphene (Darvon)

Opioids can produce side effects including mild dizziness, drowsiness, sedation and unclear thinking. Other side effects may include constipation, nausea and vomiting. Taking a stool softener or laxative may help relieve constipation. If you have trouble taking medications by mouth, some opioids are available in patch form. The medication is continuously absorbed through your skin.

Another potent painkiller is the drug tramadol (Ultram). Like an opioid, this prescription medication interferes with the transmission of pain signals. Tramadol also triggers release of natural hormones in your body that help reduce pain. Side effects are usually minor and similar to those of opioids.

**Wide-field radiation.** External beam therapy is used to treat a large portion of the body, such as the entire pelvis and both thighs.

About half the men who receive this treatment say they feel better within two days. This percentage rises as lingering radiation continues to attack the cancer. The downside, however, is that the treatment can cause listlessness. It may also cause nausea if the abdomen is treated.

**Radiofrequency ablation.** A treatment called radiofrequency ablation may provide pain relief if your cancer has spread to your bones. Radiofrequency ablation has previously been used to treat cancers of the liver and kidney. Mayo Clinic doctors have found that the procedure can provide safe, effective treatment for severe cancer-related bone pain when other treatments have failed. In radiofrequency ablation, a thin needle is inserted through the skin and guided to the cancerous tumor. An electrical current is delivered through wires called electrodes. The electrodes create intense heat, which deadens cancerous tissue and may destroy nerves in the region that carry pain from the tumor site.

## Complementary therapies

Some people find pain relief from therapies that don't involve the use of medication or radiation. These complementary practices can be used in addition to conventional pain treatments, but they're

### Be persistent

The key to adequate pain relief is working with your doctor to find an effective treatment. If the first method doesn't work, try another. Keep trying until you find a therapy that controls your pain enough so that you can rest and be comfortable.

Many people think that pain is something they have to endure — that it can't be controlled. That's not true. Effective treatments are available. It's just a matter of finding the right one. Others worry that they may appear weak if they can't handle pain on their own. This also is a misconception. Advanced prostate cancer can produce severe pain because of the way it spreads to nearby bone, including the lower spine. Seeking relief from your pain is not a sign of weakness.

more commonly used in addition to medication or radiation. They range from distracting yourself with good music to the use of acupuncture. Complementary therapies are discussed in detail in Chapter 12.

## Answers to your questions

*Can hormone therapy control prostate cancer for several years?*
Yes. Many cancers adapt and learn to grow without the presence of hormones within about one to three years. But for some men, hormone therapy can control the spread of cancer for up to 10 years.

*Will hormone therapy affect my voice or outward appearance?*
No. Both should remain the same.

*Do I need to worry about becoming addicted to painkillers?*
Many pain medications can be used effectively over many months and years without danger of addiction. In cases of advanced cancer, relief of pain, not addiction, is often a primary concern.

## Chapter 9

# Coping with complications

Prostate cancer is often a double blow. The first blow is learning that you have cancer. The second comes when you find out that treating the cancer could possibly leave you impotent or incontinent. This can be even more difficult to accept than your cancer.

Fortunately, these side effects aren't always permanent. But even when they are, they don't have to be devastating. Therapies are available to help you manage the complications of prostate treatment, so you can continue to lead a productive life.

## Controlling incontinence

Long-term incontinence after prostate cancer treatment is fairly uncommon. But when it does happen, it can be frustrating and embarrassing, and it can change your life. You may stop exercising, quit going out or even resist the urge to laugh because you're afraid of accidentally wetting yourself.

Like many men, you also may be too embarrassed to ask for help. Or, perhaps, you think incontinence is the price you have to pay for having cancer, and that you'll just have to learn to live with it. That's not true. Incontinence can often be successfully treated.

During urination, a ring of muscle around the opening at the base of your bladder, called the internal urinary sphincter, relaxes.

## Identifying the problem

One of the following tests can help diagnose the type of incontinence you have and how best to treat it.

**Cystography.** A dye is inserted into your urethra through a catheter. The dye helps enhance X-ray images of your lower urinary tract and identify an abnormality.

**Cystometrography.** A device is attached to a catheter to measure the amount of pressure in your bladder as it fills with, and then releases, water.

**Cystoscopy.** A thin tube with an attached light and lens is inserted into your urethra so that your doctor can see how well your sphincter muscle is working.

**Urinary flow rate.** It measures the speed at which urine leaves the penis.

Your bladder then contracts, pushing urine past your relaxed sphincter through your urethra. The internal sphincter's ability to function depends on pelvic floor muscles in your lower pelvis. In addition, there is an external (urethral) sphincter located within the urethra below the prostate gland that also helps control urine flow.

Treatments for prostate cancer — surgery, radiation and cryosurgery — can injure your pelvic floor muscles and the nerves that control them, producing incontinence. Often, though not always, the injury heals over weeks to months as the muscles slowly regain their strength and their ability to shut off your flow of urine.

### Types of incontinence

Urinary incontinence may be generally divided into four categories:

**Stress.** It's caused by a burst of physical activity that puts pressure on the bladder, such as lifting a heavy object, swinging a golf club, coughing, sneezing or laughing. Your weakened sphincter muscle is unable to keep urine in your bladder, and some leaks out.

**Urge.** You feel an immediate need to urinate, and you may wet yourself before you get to the bathroom. This happens when your bladder is too sensitive to the stretching that occurs as it fills with urine. It contracts prematurely, trying to expel the urine.

**Overflow.** Your bladder may not contract as it should, so you can't empty it when you urinate. Scar tissue at the base of the bladder or the narrowing of the urethra also can interfere with your urine flow and your ability to empty your bladder (see "What's a urethral stricture?"). The result is that urine builds up in the bladder and puts added pressure on the bladder muscles. You may experience frequent dribbling, and it may take you a long time to urinate. When you're done urinating, you may feel as if your bladder is still full. In severe cases, you can't urinate, even when you feel the need to go.

**Mixed.** This is a combination of two or more types of incontinence, such as stress and urge incontinence.

### Treatments for incontinence

After surgery for prostate cancer, you'll need to use a catheter for two to three weeks while swollen tissues heal. Once the catheter is

## What's a urethral stricture?

A urethral stricture is a narrowing of the urethra. It occurs in 7 percent to 17 percent of people who have a radical prostatectomy. When your prostate is removed, the upper portion of the urethra is reattached to the underside of your bladder. This restores continuity of the urinary channel, which normally is surrounded by the prostate. Sometimes, scar tissue can develop around the area where the urethra and bladder were reattached, causing the urethra to narrow.

Usually, the first line of treatment is to stretch the urethra by dilating it with a thin instrument that's inserted into the urethra. This is the simplest and safest approach.

Occasionally, the stricture needs to be opened surgically by threading a small tube and cutting tool into the urethra. In some people, these procedures must be repeated more than once because of re-narrowing.

If the stricture is severe, your doctor may suggest laser treatment to vaporize scar tissue. Conventional surgery to remove the tissue is rare and is generally recommended only when other treatments have failed.

removed, you'll probably need to wear absorbent underwear. Some products are heavily padded and bulky, designed to be worn only at home or during the night. Others are briefs, which are less bulky and can be worn as underwear. There also are pads of varying thickness that you can wear inside regular cloth underwear. Most men with incontinence regain control without requiring absorbent underwear.

Aside from protective undergarments, your doctor may suggest some of the following treatments, depending on the type of incontinence you have, its severity and the chances that it will naturally improve over time. Most men eventually see a noticeable reduction in urine leakage.

**Behavior modification.** This includes timed urination, that is, going to the bathroom according to the clock rather than waiting for the urge to go. You may start off urinating every hour or so and then build up to a longer, more acceptable interval. You may also need to avoid alcohol and caffeine, which cause you to urinate more. Reducing the amount of beverages you drink in the evening will help. For stress incontinence, crossing your legs during certain events — such as when you feel a sneeze coming — may prevent urine from leaking.

**Pelvic floor muscle exercises.** These exercises, called Kegel exercises, involve contracting and releasing your pelvic floor muscles to help improve muscle condition and tone (see "Strengthening your pelvic floor muscles" on page 109).

You want to exercise two groups of muscles — the muscles that you tighten when you want to prevent a bowel movement or hold back gas, and the muscles at the base of your penis that you use to ejaculate semen or expel the final drops of urine.

As muscle tone and strength improve, you'll gain greater control over your bladder. Kegel exercises are most effective for mild to moderate incontinence and often bring considerable improvement in about one to three months.

**Medications.** Drugs such as hyoscyamine (Cystospaz, Levsin), oxybutynin (Ditropan), and tolterodine (Detrol) help control urge incontinence by relaxing abdominal muscles and decreasing bladder contractions. You generally take the medication two to four

## Strengthening your pelvic floor muscles

It's generally best to do Kegel exercises just once or twice a day.
Performing them too often may make your muscles tired and
cause more leakage. Follow these steps:

1. Tighten those muscles you use to stop a bowel movement.
2. At the same time, tighten the muscles at the base of your
   penis. You may feel your penis pull in slightly toward
   your body.
3. Hold both sets of muscles as tightly as possible for a count
   of five.
4. Relax your muscles and rest for one minute.
5. Repeat this exercise six times.

When you're able to do the exercises easily, increase the number of repetitions to 10 and decrease the rest period between
repetitions to 10 seconds. Also, try to do the exercises in different
positions — while standing, sitting and lying down. Some men
find it helpful to do the exercises while sitting on the toilet seat.
You might also consider doing them before going to bed. This
allows your muscles to rest while you sleep.

If you have problems doing Kegel exercises, a physical
therapist may be able to help you with the use of biofeedback or
electrical stimulation. In biofeedback, electrodes that monitor
muscle contractions are placed on your skin near your pelvic
muscles. They record the strength of the contractions and
allow you to see if you're using the right muscles. Electrical
stimulation involves using mild electrical impulses to stimulate
your pelvic floor muscles to contract.

times a day, depending on how well you can tolerate it. Side effects
may include dry mouth, blurred vision and constipation.

The decongestant pseudoephedrine, used in many over-the-
counter allergy and cold medications, is sometimes recommended
for stress incontinence. It slightly tightens the urinary sphincter,
reducing leakage during episodes of pressure. However,
pseudoephedrine can produce a rapid heartbeat in some people.

Even though the medication is available without a prescription, you shouldn't use it regularly without first consulting your doctor.

**Catheters.** If your bladder can't contract forcefully enough to expel urine, you may need to practice self-catheterization. Your doctor or nurse will instruct you on how to insert a soft, narrow tube (catheter) inside your penis and thread it into your bladder. Although this sounds difficult and painful, after a few times most men lose their anxiety about the procedure and are comfortable doing it. You can carry the catheter with you. All you need is the privacy of a bathroom.

Another type of catheter is a condom catheter, worn over the penis. The condom has a tube that drains urine from the condom into a bag that you wear on your leg. These devices generally aren't recommended because they can lead to infection.

**Penile clamps.** This device clamps onto the outside of your penis, squeezing the urethra closed to prevent leakage. Clamps aren't advised because they can scar or damage the penis.

**Surgery.** If you've had leakage problems for at least a year without any sign of improvement from medicine or exercises, your doctor may suggest surgery. Several surgical procedures are available:

*Bulking agents.* The least invasive procedure involves injecting a bulking substance into the lining of your urethra at the base of your bladder to reduce leakage. The most common bulking agent is collagen, a protein found naturally in your body. The collagen used in surgery comes from cows.

During this procedure, a cystoscope is inserted into your penis and guided up to the bottom of your bladder. A needle containing the bulking substance is then threaded through the cystoscope. When the needle reaches the base of your bladder, the doctor injects the bulking substance into surrounding urethral tissues, where it puffs up the tissues and narrows the opening of your bladder.

You may need three or four injections before you notice an improvement in your bladder control. And because your body absorbs collagen, you'll probably need repeated injections.

If your incontinence is a result of radiation therapy, you may not be a good candidate for this procedure, because scar tissue caused by the radiation may prevent the bulking agent from working properly.

*Artificial sphincter.* This treatment for severe, long-term incontinence involves the implantation of a device, called an artificial sphincter, that functions like your natural sphincter. The device is an inflatable silicone cuff that's placed around the urethra or the base of your bladder. This treatment is necessary in less than 1 percent of men with incontinence.

The cuff operates a little like an arm cuff for taking blood pressure, except that it's much smaller. Instead of inflating with air, it inflates with a saline solution that's stored in a tiny reservoir in your lower abdomen. You inflate the cuff by triggering a pump implanted in your scrotum. The cuff squeezes, shutting off the flow of urine. To urinate, you deflate the cuff, allowing urine to flow out of your bladder.

Most people remain in the hospital for a few days after artificial sphincter surgery. You can't use the sphincter for about six weeks, until your urethra and bladder have had time to heal. You can damage the sphincter by sitting on a bicycle, for instance, or a horse, unless you use a special seat.

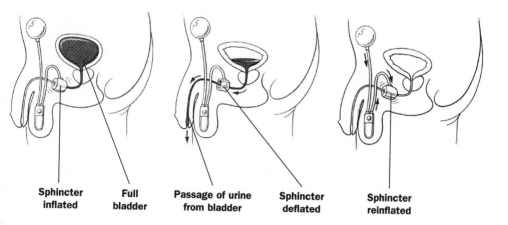

| Sphincter inflated | Full bladder | Passage of urine from bladder | Sphincter deflated | Sphincter reinflated |

An artificial sphincter uses a tiny silicone cuff placed around the urethra to treat incontinence. When inflated, the cuff squeezes the urethra, preventing urine from leaking. To urinate, you deflate the cuff, allowing urine to pass.

*Electric stimulator.* A stimulator that's implanted in your spine sends tiny electric impulses to the nerves that control your bladder. These impulses may help reduce involuntary bladder contractions that cause urge incontinence.

*Other procedures.* Sometimes it's necessary to surgically remove blockages in your urinary tract, improve the position of your bladder neck or add support to weakened pelvic muscles.

## Getting help for impotence

Impotence can result from your cancer or your treatment. As the cancer grows, it can invade and damage the nerves attached to your prostate gland that control your erections. Cancer treatment such as surgery, radiation and cryosurgery also can damage these nerves. Although hormone therapy doesn't injure the nerves, it almost completely eliminates testosterone, leaving you with no desire for sexual activity. The nerves work, but nothing stimulates them. There are three general ways to treat impotence.

### Medication
Most doctors turn first to one of the following prescription drugs:

**Sildenafil.** For some men, sildenafil (Viagra) produces remarkable results. Unfortunately, initial studies suggest that sildenafil doesn't work as well for impotence due to nerve damage as it does for other causes of impotence.

Unlike most other treatments for impotence, sildenafil produces a natural instead of an artificial erection. You still need stimulation to get an erection. The drug helps you respond to the stimulation by relaxing your smooth muscle cells, which in turn increases blood flow and makes it easier to have and maintain an erection.

You take the drug about an hour before anticipated sexual activity. The drug is effective for about four hours and shouldn't be used more than once a day. Many men are able to maintain an erection even after multiple orgasms.

Don't take sildenafil if you're also using nitrates, such as nitroglycerin. Taken together, this mix of medicine can substantially lower your blood pressure and produce a fatal heart attack.

Sildenafil can cause other side effects. The most common is facial flushing, which generally lasts no more than five to 10 minutes. You might also have a temporary mild headache or an upset stomach. Higher doses can produce short-term visual problems, including seeing a slight bluish tinge to objects, blurred vision and increased light sensitivity. These effects subside a few hours after taking the drug.

**Alprostadil.** This medication is a synthetic version of the hormone prostaglandin E. Like sildenafil, it helps relax smooth muscle tissue in the penis, which enhances blood flow and causes an erection. Sometimes, alprostadil is combined with other medications to improve its effects. Instead of taken as a pill, alprostadil is delivered one of two ways:

*Self-intraurethral therapy.* Using a disposable applicator, you insert a tiny suppository — about half the size of a grain of rice — into the tip of your penis. The brand name of this suppository is MUSE.

The suppository, placed about 2 inches into your urethra, is absorbed by erectile tissue in your penis, increasing the blood flow that causes an erection. A rubber ring placed around the base of your penis before the suppository is inserted helps trap the blood and maintain an erection.

Side effects may include some pain, dizziness and formation of hard, fibrous tissue. After a test dose in the doctor's office, you learn to do the procedure yourself.

*Self-injection.* You use a fine needle to inject alprostadil (Caverject, Edex) into the base or side of your penis. The medication needs

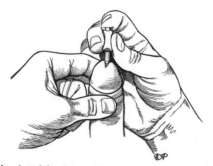

**Self-intraurethral therapy involves injecting a tiny suppository into the tip of your penis to help relax smooth muscle tissue and increase blood flow to the penis.**

to go into one of the two cylindrical, sponge-like structures that run the length of your penis on each side. Alprostadil increases blood flow into the structures, producing an erection.

It generally takes five to 20 minutes for the drug to work, with the erection lasting about an hour. Because the needle used is very thin — like needles used for diabetes and allergies — pain from the injection is usually minor.

You'll need to be careful to inject the needle along the side of your penis and not at the top or the bottom. At the top are arteries, veins and nerves, and at the bottom is the urethra. If you hit either area, you won't get an erection and you'll need to wait at least 24 hours before you can use the medication again. If this happens more than once, contact your doctor for more instruction.

Side effects may include bleeding from the injection, and on rare occasions, a prolonged, painful erection (priapism). To minimize the risk of a prolonged erection, it's important that you test the medication to determine the proper dose. If an erection continues for more than four hours, the blood trapped inside your penis becomes thick because of oxygen loss. This can damage tissue in your penis. Should you experience a prolonged erection, placing a towel-covered ice pack on the penis usually stops the erection. Taking an over-the-counter decongestant that causes your blood vessels to shrink also may relieve the condition.

If these methods don't help and the erection continues for more than four hours, call your doctor or go to an emergency room. Next time, you may need to decrease the amount of medication in order to reduce the duration of the erection.

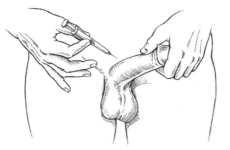

**Self-injection therapy involves injecting medication directly into a specific area of the penis to increase blood flow and cause an erection.**

Other side effects, which also are rare, may include a lump (fibrosis) where you inject the drug. It usually goes away when you stop the injections. One way to prevent fibrosis is to vary the injection site and to limit the injections to two or three times a week. Bruising of your skin also can occur if you accidentally nick a small blood vessel with the needle. To minimize bruising, keep pressure on the injection site for three to five minutes after the injection.

### Vacuum devices

This method uses vacuum pressure to draw blood into your penis. You place a plastic tube over your penis. Using a hand pump, you draw the air out of the plastic tube. As you do this, blood is pulled into the tissue of your penis, producing an erection. You then slip off an elastic ring mounted on the base of the plastic tube, pulling it onto the base of your penis. The ring traps the blood inside your penis, allowing you to keep your erection once the tube is removed. Remove the ring within 30 minutes to restore normal blood flow to your penis. If you don't, you could damage penile tissue.

Some men find the elastic ring uncomfortable and believe that it looks unnatural. In addition, your penis may feel cold because there's no blood circulation. However, a vacuum pump works in more than 90 percent of cases and doesn't require medication or surgery.

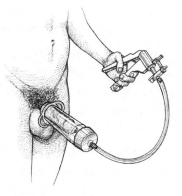

**A vacuum device uses a hand pump to draw blood into the penis and create an erection. An elastic ring placed at the base of the penis keeps it erect.**

## Penile implants

If other treatments fail or don't work well, another option to consider is a surgical implant. There are four types:

**Semirigid, bendable rod.** This is the easiest implant to use and the least likely to malfunction. Two hard, but flexible, rods made of wires and covered with silicone or polyurethane are placed inside your penis. They give you a permanent erection. You bend your penis down toward your body to hide the erection, and bend it up to have sexual intercourse.

Although it looks unnatural and takes some getting used to, this implant requires less surgical time than other implants. It has no mechanical parts to break, and it has a high success rate.

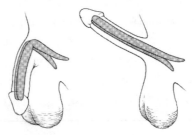

With a semirigid rod implant, the penis is always erect. To hide the erection, the implanted rods are bent down.

**Inflatable implant with pump.** This implant works more naturally than do the semirigid rods. Instead of having a permanent erection, you produce an erection only when you want one.

Two hollow cylinders are placed into your penis. These cylinders are connected to a tiny pump in your scrotum and to a reservoir in either your scrotum or your lower abdomen. When you squeeze the pump, fluid from the reservoir fills the cylinders and produces an erection.

This gives you the most natural erection of any implant. It's also the only implant that achieves the full girth of your natural erection. In addition, the device is easily concealed and very effective, but it's more likely than most other implants to undergo mechanical failure.

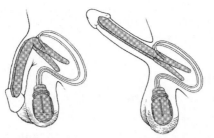

The inflatable implant with a pump includes a very small pump and a reservoir. To achieve an erection, you squeeze the pump, which causes fluid from the reservoir to fill inflatable cylinders in the penis.

**Inflatable implant without pump.** A device implanted near the head of your penis controls the flow of fluid inside cylinders implanted along the length of your penis. To get an erection, you squeeze the head of your penis. This releases fluid into the cylinders. To shift the fluid back and produce a limp penis, you bend the implant and press a release valve.

**Interlocking blocks.** This is similar to the semirigid rod implant, except that a series of small blocks connected by a steel cable is implanted into your penis. The penis doesn't become erect until you lock the blocks in place. It's simple to use and easy to conceal, and it produces an erection only when you want one.

## Dealing with bowel disorders

Approximately 5 percent to 20 percent of men who receive radiation therapy for prostate cancer experience temporary gastrointestinal problems. These may include blood in the stool, cramps, rectal irritation and discharge, diarrhea, or a sense of having to use the bathroom immediately.

External beam therapy is accurate in targeting prostate cancer, but your rectum also usually receives some radiation. The most common side effect of this is rectal irritation. In most cases, no radiation is given to the intestines. Injury from radiation that requires surgical repair is rare, happening less than 1 percent of the time.

Prostate surgery also can cause rectal injury. However, this too is rare. If there's an injury, it's usually repaired during the surgery with no permanent damage.

Bowel disorders can continue for several months after treatment. Most improve on their own.

### Blood in the stool

Radiation therapy can injure the lining of your rectum. One result may be abnormal growth of tiny blood vessels near the surface that bleed easily. Sometimes the bleeding can continue for years.

Treatment depends on the severity of the bleeding. Often, the first step is to monitor the bleeding to see if you're passing only small amounts of blood. If the bleeding is moderate to heavy, your doctor may prescribe stool softeners or medicated enemas to reduce pressure on your rectal lining as stool passes. For severe cases, laser therapy can often destroy the vessels causing the bleeding.

### Diarrhea

Diarrhea may result from radiation, but usually only in cases in which it's necessary to treat the pelvis. Generally, its effects are temporary. Over-the-counter antidiarrheal medications such as Imodium, Kaopectate or Pepto-Bismol may help reduce your symptoms.

To prevent dehydration during episodes of diarrhea, drink at least eight glasses of clear liquids a day, including water or clear sodas. Avoid dairy products, caffeine, and fatty or highly seasoned foods, which can prolong diarrhea. Signs of dehydration include excessive thirst, dry mouth, weakness, dark-colored urine and little or no urination.

### Constipation

Medications used to treat prostate cancer may reduce the normal activity of your bowels. When this happens, fecal material becomes packed and hard, producing cramps and constipation. In some instances, you can relieve constipation by following a regular eating schedule and including high-fiber foods, such as whole-grain cereals and breads, fresh vegetables and fresh fruits. Add these to your diet gradually to avoid possible discomfort caused by gas. Exercising daily and drinking plenty of fluids also will help reduce constipation.

You may want to try a natural fiber supplement, such as Citrucel, Fiberall or Metamucil. It should help within one to three days. Fiber supplements are generally safe, but because they're so absorbent, make sure to take them with plenty of water. Otherwise, they can become constipating — the opposite of what you want them to do.

If these measures don't help, ask your doctor about use of a stool softener or a laxative. There are several types:

**Stool softeners.** These are the most gentle products. They're sold over the counter under a variety of brand names, including Colace, Correctol and Surfak. Mineral oil shouldn't be taken as a stool softener because it can block absorption of key vitamins.

**Saline laxatives.** This includes the over-the-counter product Phillips' Milk of Magnesia, which works by increasing water content in your stool.

**Stimulant laxatives.** These are the most powerful and should be taken only when other measures fail to induce a bowel movement. Over-the-counter brand names include Dulcolax, Ex-Lax and Senokot.

## Answers to your questions

*How long can I expect to wear absorbent underwear after treatment?*
The length of time varies. One to four months isn't unusual.

*What's the difference between impotence and erectile dysfunction?*
The terms are often used interchangeably, but they aren't exactly the same. Impotence means that your penis is unable to become firm (erect) or stay firm long enough to have sexual intercourse. Erectile dysfunction includes impotence, plus other abnormalities, such as prolonged erection or abnormal curvature of the penis.

*If I have good erections before treatment, does that increase the chance I'll be able to have normal erections afterward?*
Yes. Younger, healthier men experiencing strong erections are far more likely to continue normal erections after treatment than are older men or men already having erectile problems.

*Are treatments for incontinence and impotence covered by Medicare?*
Most are. However, Medicare may not pay the entire cost,
especially for medications. You may have to pay a portion of
the cost yourself.

## Chapter 10

# Getting on with life

There's no doubt prostate cancer can change your life. Day in and day out, it can dominate your thinking and actions — upsetting your daily routine, straining your emotions and eroding your relationships.

But it doesn't have to. Armed with insights from health care professionals and those who've been through it, you can learn to cope with cancer and minimize its effects. There is life after treatment for prostate cancer, and that life can be enjoyable.

## Preparing for follow-up visits

Some men dread going in for checkups. This is natural. But try to balance your worries with positive thoughts. Keep in mind that the treatment you've received, and continue to receive, is good. Ask plenty of questions during your first few follow-up visits, such as how frequently you'll need checkups and what tests you'll receive.

At first, you may need to see your doctor every three months. Eventually, your visits may spread out to once or twice a year. In addition to a physical exam, each checkup may include X-rays and a prostate-specific antigen (PSA) test to help determine whether the cancer has returned or progressed.

## Questions for your doctor

If you have questions about what to expect after treatment for prostate cancer — even if they seem embarrassing or dumb — discuss them with your doctor. Here are 10 question get you started:

1. "How often will I need a checkup?"
2. "What will my checkups consist of, and will they always be the same?"
3. "What are some signs that my cancer has returned or progressed?"
4. "How likely are these signs or symptoms to occur?"
5. "What changes might I see that are OK — that aren't danger signs?"
6. "Should I change my diet?"
7. "Do I need to alter my daily routine?"
8." If I experience pain, what should I do?"
9. "What's the best way for me to get in touch with you if I have questions or concerns?"
10. "Is there someone else I can talk to if you aren't available?"

Adapted from: "Facing Forward: A Guide for Cancer Survivors," National Cancer Institute, National Institutes of Health, 2002

## Overcoming cancer's emotional toll

There's no right way to act or feel if you have cancer. The disease can produce a roller coaster of emotions that vary from person to person. What's important is that you recognize and accept your actions and emotions and find healthy ways to deal with them.

### What you can expect

Here are feelings that may accompany prostate cancer treatment.

**Anxiety.** If you experience side effects from your treatment, such as impotence or incontinence, talking about them, as well as the cancer, may embarrass you.

Impotence or incontinence can also undermine your self-confidence. You may withdraw from social and business gatherings because you're afraid of embarrassing yourself. This can be difficult to overcome if you've been self-confident.

**Emptiness.** If you've had surgery to remove your prostate, you may feel a void that's hard to describe, especially if the surgery has caused impotence. You might sense a loss of maleness. You may feel as if you're less of a man, just as some women may feel they're less feminine after a hysterectomy or breast removal.

Treatment for prostate cancer can reduce or eliminate production of male hormones, mainly testosterone. This can affect how you respond to sexual stimulation. It might be more difficult to have or maintain an erection. Fortunately, many treatments for impotence are available.

**Depression.** Depression is common among people with cancer. You may grow deeply sad and discouraged over what has happened to you. You may even become pessimistic about your future. These feelings may last for only a short time, they may come and go, or they may linger for weeks or months.

Depression that lingers can interfere with your ability to manage your life. It can precipitate a downward spiral that can make you more and more miserable. Because you're depressed, you don't put any effort into coping with your daily problems. And when the problems get worse, so does your depression.

A person with depression may have some, most, or all of these signs and symptoms:

- Lasting sadness
- Loss of interest or pleasure in most activities
- Neglect of personal responsibilities and personal care
- Irritability and mood swings
- Change in appetite, and weight gain or loss
- Recurrent morning awakenings or other changes in sleep patterns
- Feelings of restlessness
- Feelings of hopelessness or helplessness
- Extreme fatigue, loss of energy, or slowed movements
- Continuous negative view of the world and others
- Feelings of worthlessness and inappropriate feelings of guilt
- Decreased concentration, attention and memory

- Increased focus on physical complaints
- Thoughts of death or suicide

Depression must be professionally treated. More than 80 percent of people who seek treatment show improvement in symptoms within a matter of weeks. However, many people don't receive treatment because they're unaware of their condition or they don't view depression as a serious health problem. Instead, they think they can handle the condition on their own.

**What you can do**

The following strategies can help you cope with some of the difficulties of cancer:

**Be prepared.** Ask your doctor questions and read about prostate cancer and its potential side effects. The fewer the surprises, the more quickly you'll adapt.

**Maintain as normal a routine as you can.** Don't let the cancer or side effects from treatment dominate your day. Try to follow the routine and lifestyle you had before learning of your cancer. Go back to work, take a trip, join your children or grandchildren on an outing. You'll do better if you engage in activities that give you a sense of purpose, fulfillment and meaning. But realize that to begin with, you may have some limitations. Start slowly and gradually build your level of endurance.

**Try not to wallow in sad feelings.** Although depression requires professional treatment, you may simply have the blues. Seek diversions and plan at least one enjoyable experience every day. This might include a hobby, playing golf, or going to a movie. Make it something you enjoy and look forward to.

**Get plenty of exercise.** Exercise helps fight depression and is a good way to relieve tension and frustration.

**Look for ways to compensate.** If you have problems with incontinence, sit in the back of the movie theater or meeting room instead of the front. That way you'll be nearer to a bathroom if you need one. Sit in an aisle seat on an airplane, train or bus. Wear absorbent undergarments if you're not sure whether you'll be near a bathroom. Avoid caffeinated products and alcohol because they increase urination.

**Open up to a friend, family member or counselor.** Cancer is too heavy a load to carry all by yourself. Sometimes it helps to talk with someone about your deepest feelings and fears. Your mind and body aren't separate. The better you feel emotionally, the better you're physically able to cope with your illness.

**Don't avoid sexual contact.** Your natural reaction to impotence may be to avoid all sexual contact. Don't fall for this feeling. Touching, holding, hugging and caressing may become far more important to you and your partner. In fact, the closeness you develop in these actions can produce greater sexual intimacy than you've ever had before. There are many ways to express your sexuality.

**Look for the positive.** Cancer doesn't have to be all negative. Good can come out of it. Confrontation with cancer may lead you to grow emotionally and spiritually, identify what really matters to you, settle long-standing disputes, and spend more time with people important to you.

## Regaining your strength

Fatigue is a common side effect of prostate cancer and treatment. It can be a frustrating obstacle when you're struggling to keep a normal schedule and maintain a good quality of life. Fatigue may result for any number of reasons:
- Stress and depression over your diagnosis
- Difficulty sleeping
- Surgery or radiation therapy
- Metabolic abnormalities related to the cancer or its treatment
- Low red blood cell count (anemia) from the cancer or its treatment

### Self-care for fatigue
To help reduce fatigue, follow these steps:

**Tell your doctor.** Don't hide your fatigue or try to ignore it. There may be a physical cause, such as anemia, that can be treated.

**Rest.** Don't fight fatigue. If you need short naps during the day, take them.

## Spirituality and healing

Spiritual peace can be a powerful healing force. Spirituality is often confused with religion. But spirituality isn't so much connected to a specific belief or form of worship as it is with the spirit or the soul. Spirituality is about meaning, values and purpose in life.

Religion may be one way of expressing spirituality, but it's not the only way. For some people, spirituality is feeling in tune with nature and the universe. For others, spirituality is expressed through music, meditation or art.

Numerous studies have attempted to measure the effect of spirituality on illness and recovery. In reviewing many of these studies, researchers at Georgetown University School of Medicine found that at least 80 percent of studies suggest that spiritual beliefs have a beneficial effect on health. The researchers concluded that people who consider themselves to be spiritual enjoy better health, live longer, recover from illness more quickly and with fewer complications, suffer less depression and chemical addiction, have lower blood pressure, and cope better with serious disease, including cancer.

No one knows exactly how spirituality affects health. Some experts attribute the healing effect to hope, which is known to benefit your immune system. Others liken spiritual acts and beliefs to meditation, which decreases muscle tension and can lower your heart rate. Still others point to the social connectedness spirituality often provides.

An important point to keep in mind is that although spirituality is associated with healing and better health, it isn't a cure. Spirituality can help you live more fully despite your symptoms, but no studies have found that it actually cures health problems. It's best to view spirituality as a helpful healing force — as a supplement to, but not a substitute for, traditional medical care.

**Set reasonable goals.** Take one day at a time and try not to overdo it. But don't sit back and do nothing, either. Inactivity also produces fatigue.

**Delegate chores.** You may need to ask others to do tasks you've traditionally done, such as cutting the grass or shoveling snow.

**Practice relaxation techniques.** Wrestling with heavy emotions, such as anxiety and fear, can contribute to your fatigue. Talk with your doctor, a nurse or a counselor about stress reduction techniques, and which ones might work best for you (see "Simple ways to relax" on page 128).

**Try to get a good night's sleep.** Here are some suggestions that can help you sleep better:

- Get in the habit of going to bed and waking up at the same time each day. This helps program your body to follow an established sleep cycle.
- Develop a nightly routine before getting into bed. Perhaps it's reading a book, taking a warm bath or relaxing in front of the television. This sends messages to your body that it's almost time for bed.
- Avoid foods and beverages that can disrupt your sleep. Anything with caffeine, such as coffee or chocolate, can make it more difficult for you to fall asleep. Alcoholic drinks may help you fall asleep, but they can disrupt your sleep patterns and keep you from getting the deep sleep you need.
- Try to get at least 30 minutes of physical activity daily, preferably five to six hours before you go to bed, and keep active during the day. This helps you to sleep better at night.
- During the night, close your door or create a subtle background noise, such as a fan, to drown out other noises. Keep your bedroom temperature comfortable and drink fewer beverages before bed so that you won't have to get up as often during the night to urinate.

## Eating better to feel better

A nutritious diet provides the fuel that lets your body maintain its strength and operate at its best. That's why a nutritious diet is especially important if you're undergoing treatment for cancer. If you don't eat enough food or the right kinds of foods, your body resorts to using stored nutrients. This may weaken your natural

## Simple ways to relax

Relaxation helps relieve stress that can make it difficult for you to concentrate, sleep or recover. There are many ways to relax. Here are some techniques you can try:

**Deep breathing.** Deep breathing from your diaphragm is more relaxing than breathing from your chest. It also exchanges more carbon dioxide for oxygen, giving you more energy. To practice deep breathing:

1. Sit comfortably with your feet flat on the floor.
2. Loosen tight clothing around your abdomen and waist.
3. Place your hands in your lap or at your sides.
4. Close your eyes if it helps you to relax.
5. Breathe in slowly through your nose while counting to four. Allow your abdomen to expand as you breathe in.
6. Pause for a second and then exhale at a normal rate through your mouth.
7. Repeat until you feel more relaxed.

**Progressive muscle relaxation.** This technique involves relaxing a series of muscles one at a time. First, raise the tension level in a group of muscles, such as a leg or arm, by tightening the muscles and then slowly relaxing them. Concentrate on letting the tension go in each muscle. Then move on to the next muscle group.

**Word repetition.** Choose a word or phrase that's a cue for you to relax, and then constantly repeat it. While repeating the word or phrase, try to breathe deeply and slowly and think of something that gives you pleasant sensations of warmth and heaviness.

**Guided imagery.** Lie quietly and picture yourself in a pleasant and peaceful setting. Experience the setting with all of your senses, as if you were actually there. For instance, imagine lying on a beach. Picture the beautiful blue sky, smell the salt water, hear the waves, and feel the warm breeze on your skin. The messages your brain gets help calm and relax you.

defenses against infection. The better you eat, the more able you may be to handle chemotherapy or radiation therapy treatments.

When you're being treated for cancer, what you eat and how often you eat may be different from when you're healthy. Normally, nutrition recommendations stress eating plenty of fruits, vegetables and grains, and cutting back on fat and sugar. For people undergoing treatment for cancer, however, appetite can be a problem. Eating high-calorie foods can promote energy. Ensuring that you eat adequate protein-containing foods can promote strength and help repair body tissues. Since it's important to eat nutritiously, the following tips might help you plan meals and snacks that make every bite count.

**Increase calories.** During treatment and recovery, your need for calories may be greater than usual. Maintaining your weight is a helpful sign that you're eating enough. Add calories by:

- Using butter, margarine, mayonnaise, oil, cream cheese, gravies, sauces, salad dressings, sour cream, whipping cream and other fatty spreads or toppings. Spread on breads, vegetables, chicken, fish and seafood. Use whipping cream in cooked cereals, soups, mashed potatoes, or to top fruits and desserts. Sauteed or fried foods are higher in calories than are baked, broiled or steamed items.
- Topping foods with sugar, jam, jelly and honey. Sugar-sweetened cereals and granola and sweetened fresh and canned fruit and juices are higher in calories than are their unsweetened counterparts. Dried fruit also is a calorie-packed nutritious snack.
- Drinking beverages with calories — fruit juices, lemonade, soft drinks and fortified fruit drinks. Add sugar or cream to coffee and tea.

**Ensure adequate protein.** Eating adequate amounts of protein doesn't necessarily mean eating large amounts of meat. Other options include:

- About 2 to 3 ounces of poultry, fish or shellfish for a meal. Think of these foods as condiments rather than the main course. Use them into casseroles, pasta dishes and stir-fries.

- Foods such as beans and tofu are high in protein and can stand in for meat. Soy in tofu may make cancer cells more vulnerable to radiation.
- Eggs — fried, scrambled, hard-boiled or an omelet — can make a healthy meal. Eggs can also be used in custards, sandwich fillings and french toast.
- Small amounts of cheese served along with crackers, added to sandwiches, or melted onto vegetables or pasta. A half cup of cottage cheese with fruit also is a healthy snack.
- Milk and milk products. Because of the controversy over the possible role of calcium in prostate cancer, try to keep milk and yogurt consumption — products especially high in calcium — to no more than 2 cups daily to help ensure adequate protein intake.

**Stock up on nutritional drinks.** These products, available as a liquid or powder, are sold under brand names such as Ensure, Sustacal, Boost and Carnation Instant Breakfast. The drinks are high in calories and protein, and they contain extra vitamins and minerals.

---

### What about all those nutrition pills?

Should I take a vitamin, mineral or herbal pill? Can it help fight my cancer? The answer to both questions, generally, is no.

People who eat well during cancer treatment are better able to cope with their disease and the side effects of treatment. However, there's no scientific evidence that a vitamin, mineral or herbal supplement can cure cancer or help you better withstand treatment.

The National Cancer Institute recommends that you get your vitamins, minerals and other nutrients from foods or beverages, not individual supplements. Too much of some vitamins or minerals can be as dangerous as too little. Large doses of some vitamins, minerals and herbs may even interfere with your cancer treatment, and keep it from working as it should. Don't take any supplements without first talking with your doctor or a registered dietitian.

Nutritional drinks can be used as meal substitutes if you don't feel like eating. You also can drink them between meals to improve your diet and give you added calories, protein and other nutrients. Because the drinks need no refrigeration, you can carry them with you and have them whenever you feel hungry or thirsty. They can also be chilled.

Some people find nutritional products difficult to drink because they don't care for their flavor or texture. If this is true for you, try this simple recipe and see if it improves the product's appeal: Combine one can of a liquid drink with a piece of fruit or a scoop of ice cream. Blend the mixture in a blender and serve it over ice.

If you're not certain whether you could benefit from a nutritional drink, talk with your doctor or a registered dietitian.

### Stimulating your appetite during chemotherapy

Loss of appetite is common when you're ill or recovering from an illness. The nausea and vomiting that you may experience during chemotherapy can make food unappealing. To improve your diet and stimulate your appetite:

**Eat whenever you feel hungry.** You may be used to eating three meals a day. But when you're fighting cancer, you can't afford to limit yourself to this restrictive schedule. If your appetite and taste buds seem in disarray, eating smaller meals throughout the day may work better for you. Taking just a few bites of the right food or a few sips of a nutritious drink every hour or so can help a lot. Ordinarily, people shouldn't eat at bedtime. But if you can eat something before going to bed, do it.

**Prepare and freeze meals ahead of time.** This allows you to have something quick and easy to fix on days when you don't feel like cooking.

**Choose foods that look and smell good.** Some cancer treatments can change your sense of taste and smell. So if red meat is unappetizing, try other sources of protein such as chicken, fish, eggs or dairy products.

Most people with cancer find soups and soft foods are the easiest to eat and digest. Experiment with lightly seasoned dishes made with eggs, poultry and pasta. These dishes are generally well tolerated.

**Try new foods.** Some foods you used to love may now taste bad. On the other hand, foods you used to avoid you may now find more appealing.

**Don't force yourself to eat your favorite foods.** Especially when you're nauseated, avoid those foods you like the best. Trying to eat them may leave you with a permanent distaste for these items, and you may forever link them with unpleasant side effects. Consider saving your favorites for when you're feeling well.

**Enhance the flavor.** You may find food tastes bland. Try small amounts of seasoning. You can also try marinating poultry and meat in fruit juices, sweet wine, if permitted, or sauces.

**Drink less with meals.** Beverages are important. Aim for 6 to 8 cups of fluids daily. But try to limit beverages at mealtimes because they can make you feel full when you're not. Instead, save them for the end of the meal.

**Change the atmosphere.** Eating in a different setting may stimulate your appetite. Invite a friend over, play music, light some candles, or watch a video or favorite television program.

If you still have trouble eating a few weeks after your treatment, ask your doctor for advice. A registered dietitian who specializes in helping people with cancer can devise an eating plan that's suited to your tastes and unique nutritional needs.

## Going back to work

Having cancer doesn't mean your career is ruined or that you'll never again pull your weight at work. In fact, the vast majority of people with cancer return to work. And surveys show that people who have been treated for cancer are just as productive as other workers, and no more likely to take sick days.

Your job is an important part of your life, providing personal fulfillment, income, enjoyment and a sense of contributing to the community. It can also become a place of rehabilitation and uplifting therapy, especially if you're treated as a valuable member of the team. Many men with prostate cancer find that getting back to

## Curbing nausea and diarrhea

Radiation, medications and anxiety all may contribute to nausea and diarrhea. Here are some practical suggestions to help you combat these conditions:

### Nausea

- Stock your refrigerator and cupboards with soothing foods, such as clear sodas, soups and crackers.
- Eat something dry, such as a piece of toast or saltine crackers, right after you wake up.
- Eat salty foods rather than sweet ones.
- Avoid hot, greasy, spicy or strong-smelling foods.
- After you've eaten, sit up for 10 to 20 minutes and let your food settle.

### Diarrhea

- Drink plenty of clear fluids.
- Eat small amounts of food throughout the day instead of three large meals.
- Eat foods and drink liquids that contain potassium and sodium, two important minerals often lost during diarrhea. High-sodium liquids include bouillon and broth. Foods and beverages high in potassium include bananas, peach or apricot nectar, and boiled or mashed potatoes. Sports drinks contain high levels of both sodium and potassium.
- Avoid greasy foods, foods with skins or seeds, and gas-forming vegetables, such as broccoli, cabbage and cauliflower.
- Try these foods: yogurt, cottage cheese, rice, noodles, warm cereal, smooth peanut butter and white bread, skinless chicken or turkey, and lean beef.

work helps them regain a sense of normality in their lives. At first, you may need to make a few adjustments. But eventually you should be able to resume your regular schedule and activities. Before you return to work:

- Talk with your doctor about how much you should work. It's often best to ease back into your work schedule.

- Talk with your supervisor about adjusting your hours or duties when you first return.
- Consider how you'll respond to co-workers who may have questions about your cancer and how you're doing. Practicing what you're going to say ahead of time can make the interchange more comfortable.

## Communicating with family and friends

Cancer has a way of stifling communication when you need it the most. Family members may find it difficult to come to grips with your illness, so they aren't able to talk with you about important issues. And well-meaning friends — not knowing what to say or do, and not wanting to upset you — may steer clear of conversations about your health. They may even spend less time with you.

Here are some ways you can make it easier for family and friends to give you needed support:

**Accept the emotional timetable of your loved ones.** You may want to talk about important issues related to your illness before some of your family and friends are ready. Interpret their body

### Getting your life in order

A common response to a diagnosis of cancer — even when the prognosis is good — is to organize your life. You may feel a need to review insurance policies, update your will, or clean out the attic and give away items you no longer need.

This is understandable. Cancer makes you think about life — what's really important, what you want to achieve, and if you should die, how you can make things easier for your family. Planning for the future is good. It can save hardships and disagreements later on. But be prepared that your family may view your actions with concern. They may feel you've lost all hope and that you're giving up. Taking time to talk with family members about what you're doing and why may help alleviate their anxiety.

language, such as whether they make eye contact. If they aren't ready to talk, give them a little more time to adjust.

Just the opposite, if some of your loved ones are ready to talk before you are, postpone the discussion without hurting the person's feelings. For instance, you could say, "I know you care about this, and we need to make some decisions. But I'm not ready to talk about it yet. I really need a little more time."

Not all families are open and sharing. You or a family member may be very private and find it difficult to discuss feelings. Sometimes, it's easier to open up to someone outside your immediate circle of family and friends, such as a counselor or someone else who has had cancer.

**Call or visit family and friends.** You may think it should be the other way around. And with some of your closest family and friends it will be. They'll come to you. But try to remember people you knew who were ill and how hard it was for you to think of what to say or do to help them.

Think of ways to put family and friends at ease. Ask a busy friend what projects he has going. Invite a friend who's not a great talker to help you with a chore, such as cleaning out the garage. For friends who have plenty of their own problems, ask how things are going.

**Accept help from others and don't be afraid to ask for it.** There are times when it's crucial to work together. Fighting cancer is such a time. It's difficult to fight cancer alone. Many times your family and friends are waiting for clues as to how they can help. When they say, "Let me know if there's anything I can do for you," go ahead and tell them. Most family and friends are grateful to have a chance to show you, in practical ways, that they care. Often, all they need is an icebreaker invitation from you.

## Joining a support group

Not everyone needs a support group. Having family and friends may be all the support you need. But some may find it helpful to have people they can turn to outside their immediate circles. In general, support groups fall into two main categories — those led by health care professionals, such as a psychologist or nurse, and those led by support group members. Some are more educational and structured, and may include discussions on new treatments. Others emphasize emotional support and shared experiences. Some focus on one type of cancer, such as prostate cancer. Others include people with all types of cancer.

In addition, the Internet offers online virtual support groups, in which you can converse with others and receive updates on the latest cancer treatments via your computer. Be careful, however, about the reliability of information you find with online support groups. Although they can be excellent sources of practical advice, you also can encounter less than accurate, if not potentially harmful, information. Avoid any group that promises a cure for cancer or suggests that support groups are a cure or a substitute for medical treatment. Instead, look for groups affiliated with a reputable organization, or hosted by a medical expert.

No matter how the group is set up, the goal should be the same — to help people cope and live well with cancer.

### What support groups offer

Benefits of support groups include:

**A sense of belonging, of fitting in.** There's a special bond among people whose lives have been disrupted by the same problem. You share a sense of camaraderie. Once you experience how others accept you just as you are, you begin to feel more accepting of yourself.

**People who understand what you're going through.** Compassionate family, friends and doctors can sympathize with your problems, but they haven't experienced what you have.

People with cancer share many common threads. Support group members have a good idea of what you're feeling and experiencing. Because of this, you feel freer to express your feelings without fear that you'll hurt someone's feelings or be misunderstood.

**Exchange of advice.** You may be skeptical of some of the advice well-meaning friends give you, because they haven't had cancer. But when veteran group members talk, you know they speak with the voice of first-hand experience. They can tell you about coping

## Is a support group right for you?

If you answer yes to most of the following questions, joining a cancer support group may be a positive step for you:

- Are you comfortable sharing your feelings with others in a similar situation?
- Are you interested in hearing how others feel about their personal experiences?
- Could you benefit from the advice of others who have gone through cancer treatment?
- Do you enjoy being part of a group?
- Do you have helpful information or hints to share with others?
- Would reaching out to help others with cancer give you satisfaction?
- Would you feel comfortable around others who may have different ways of dealing with their cancer?
- Are you interested in learning more about cancer issues?

Adapted from: "Facing Forward: A Guide for Cancer Survivors," National Cancer Institute, National Institutes of Health, 2002

techniques that have worked for them and those that haven't helped.

**Opportunity to make new friends.** These friends can bring joy into your life as well as practical support — a listening ear when you need to talk, a chauffeur when you could use a relaxing drive, and a companion to exercise with.

### When support groups aren't the answer

Support groups aren't for everyone. To gain the most benefit from a group setting, you need to find the meetings enjoyable and helpful. If you find them uncomfortable, trust your instinct and stop attending the meetings.

In addition, not all support groups are beneficial. You want to be in a group where the mood is optimistic and the message positive. Some groups that aren't carefully monitored can become a place to vent and share only negative feelings that breed on themselves. This can leave you depressed and add to your frustration.

## Coping with survival

Traditionally, a cancer survivor is someone in whom there's no evidence of active disease five years after treatment. Despite the relief of winning the battle, survival can bring other emotional challenges.

During cancer treatment and recovery, relationships with family and friends may have centered on your illness. Learning to refocus those relationships on other matters and a future together can take a new way of thinking. Reclaiming your place in your family and circle of friends may be difficult at first. Tell others how you feel and openly address their fears and questions.

Many of the old stigmas associated with cancer still exist. For example, you may have to remind friends and co-workers that cancer isn't contagious and that research shows cancer survivors are just as productive as people without cancer.

There are also financial realities, such as insurance. If you experience difficulties switching or obtaining insurance, find out if your state provides health insurance for people who are difficult to insure. Look into group insurance options through professional, fraternal or political organizations.

Life after cancer can sometimes mean discarding old fears and uncertainties and facing new challenges. But as you adapt to these changes, you'll undoubtedly experience a sense of recovery and control.

The great disadvantage of online support groups is that you don't know much about who else is online with you or whether you can believe everything that's shared.

### Finding a support group

What support group you choose may depend largely on what's available in your area. To find a group:

- Ask your doctor, nurse, or other health care professional for assistance.

- Look in your telephone book or check your newspaper for a listing of support resources.
- Contact community centers, libraries or religious organizations.
- Ask others you know who have or who had cancer.
- Contact a national cancer organization such as the American Cancer Society at (800) ACS-2345, or (800) 227-2345, or Cancer Care at (800) 813-HOPE, or (800) 813-4673.

Most support groups are free, collect voluntary donations or charge only modest membership dues to cover expenses.

## Answers to your questions

*What if, months after treatment, a PSA test produces an elevated reading? Does this mean the cancer is back?*
If you still have your prostate gland, an elevated PSA level can be normal or it may indicate that the cancer is progressing. Elevated PSA levels after removal of the prostate usually indicate that cancer is present.

*How long will it take after surgery before I can exercise and take part in sporting activities again?*
Fatigue can linger for three to six months after surgery. Your ability to participate also depends on the activity and your physical condition before surgery. Somewhere between six weeks and two months after surgery you may be able to jog, golf, swim or play tennis at a leisurely pace. It may be many months, however, before you can ride a bicycle or a horse. A bicycle seat or a saddle places pressure on the lower pelvis, the location of the surgery.

*What's a living will?*
A living will is also referred to as an advance directive. It's a legal document that states your wishes about your medical care in case of a terminal illness. For example, it states whether you want to be placed on a breathing device (ventilator) or have a feeding tube. If you choose to prepare a living will, it's important that people in charge of your care, such as your doctor and a family member, receive copies.

*Does the fear that the cancer will return ever go away?*
Some people who have had successful treatment are able to get past this fear. Others aren't. But in most cases, the fear wanes as the months and years pass. No one expects you to forget you've had cancer. But your fears will become fewer and farther between as you fill your mind and time with other thoughts and activities.

# Part 4

*Prostate health*

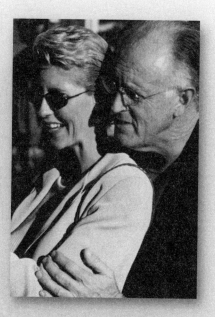

## Chapter 11

# Can you prevent prostate disease?

A lthough common, prostate problems aren't inevitable. True, there isn't any formula that can guarantee you won't get prostate disease. But there are things you can do to reduce your risk, or possibly slow the disease's progression. The three most important steps you can take to maintain prostate health — and health in general — are to eat well, keep physically active and see your doctor regularly.

## Eat more of these potential cancer fighters

The foods that you eat and the beverages that you drink may reduce your risk of prostate disease, especially cancer. Researchers are finding that certain plant-based products appear to be beneficial in preventing or controlling prostate cancer. It's not necessary that you eat these foods every day, but it may be a good idea to make these products a frequent part of your diet.

### Tomatoes and tomato products
They contain the chemical lycopene (LY-ko-pene), which gives them their red color. Lycopene is also thought to be a potent antioxidant. Antioxidants are substances that protect cells from the effects of free radicals, toxic molecules that can damage your cells.

Studies have shown that frequent consumption of tomato products or other lycopene-rich foods is associated with lower risk of prostate cancer. Lycopene found in cooked tomato products — soups, and sauces used in spaghetti and pizza — appears to provide greater cancer protection than does lycopene in raw products, such as fresh tomatoes or tomato juice. One reason may be that it's easier for your body to absorb lycopene from tomatoes after they've been cooked.

Other studies suggest that lycopene may also reduce your risk of colon, rectal, breast, lung and stomach cancers, as well as a heart attack. Watermelon and pink grapefruit and two tropical fruits — guava and pineapple — also contain small quantities of lycopene.

### Soy

Soy products come from the soybean, a legume native to northern China, and now commonly grown in the United States. Certain compounds in soy (isoflavones) appear to stimulate your body's binding proteins (globulins) that keep the sex hormones testosterone and estrogen in check. When bound, the hormones exert less effect. Because prostate cancer feeds off testosterone, researchers theorize that the less effect it has, the lower your risk is of cancer development and progression.

In Asia, where soy is a food staple, certain types of cancer, including prostate and breast cancers, are less common. However, it's uncertain whether soy or some other aspect of the Asian diet or lifestyle is responsible.

In addition to controlling cancer, there's some evidence soy may lower your risk of benign prostatic hyperplasia (BPH). It may also help reduce cholesterol levels.

### Green tea

Green tea contains a natural substance, called epigallocatechin gallate (EGCG), that's similar to substances found in vegetables and red wine. Like other anticancer agents, EGCG appears to inhibit enzyme activity necessary for cancer growth. In 1998, Mayo Clinic researchers found that low concentrations of EGCG inhibited cancer cell growth in test tubes, and at high concentrations, EGCG killed cancer cells.

## Sources of soy

Soy isn't a common ingredient in foods, but you can find items containing soy in well-stocked grocery and health food stores. Here are some items to look for:

**Soybeans.** Soak them overnight and then cook them for 2.5 hours to soften. Soybeans also come precooked (refrigerated, frozen or vacuum-packed). Add the beans to your favorite recipes, including soups, chilis, stir-fries or salads.

**Tofu.** Its neutral taste and spongy texture make it ideal for absorbing other flavors. Use it in place of meat. Tofu also comes in a silken consistency, which can be added to creamy soups or substituted for ingredients such as sour cream or mayonnaise.

**Tempeh and miso.** Both are made of fermented soybeans. Tempeh is available in a thin cake, and miso is a paste. They can be used in soups and salads or as a meat substitute.

**Textured soy protein (TSP).** Available in the frozen-food section, TSP looks like browned meat and can be used in casseroles or foods such as tacos. TSP is also found in soy burgers.

**Soy milk.** Use it in recipes or on cereal.

**Soy flour.** In baked goods, substitute soy flour for a portion of all-purpose flour. Place 2 tablespoons of soy flour in a 1-cup measuring cup and then fill the remainder of the cup with all-purpose flour. You also can substitute 1 tablespoon of soy flour and 1 to 2 tablespoons of water for each egg in baking recipes.

However, a Mayo Clinic study published in 2003 found no evidence that green tea helped men with advanced prostate cancer whose cancer had become resistant to hormone therapy. In fact, the majority of men in the study experienced side effects including nausea, vomiting, diarrhea, insomnia and confusion while consuming the equivalent of six to 12 glasses of green tea daily. Researchers said that more study is needed to determine whether green tea may be useful in treating other stages of the disease.

### Cruciferous vegetables

Cruciferous vegetables belong to the cabbage and mustard family, and include bok choy, broccoli, brussels sprouts, cabbage, cauliflower, collards, rutabagas and turnips. These vegetables contain certain chemicals that appear to block the effects of cancer-causing substances.

## Vitamins and minerals

Much of the research on the role of vitamins and minerals in preventing prostate cancer is inconclusive. Several studies have examined whether vitamins C, D, E and the mineral selenium help prevent prostate disease. Selenium, a trace element found in many foods, strengthens the antioxidant effects of vitamin E. Some studies suggest that these nutrients may reduce your risk of prostate cancer. Other studies indicate they don't provide any benefit. Current studies may provide more information on what role, if any, specific vitamins or minerals play in keeping your prostate healthy.

Researchers also are investigating the effects of the mineral zinc on prostate health. Zinc is most abundant in meat, seafood, poultry and whole grains. The prostate gland contains more zinc than does any other organ, and research suggests that too little zinc may contribute to prostate disease. In some men, taking a daily zinc supplement may shrink the prostate gland and relieve benign prostatic hyperplasia (BPH) symptoms. Zinc may also reduce inflammation associated with chronic prostatitis. However, it's not known yet how much zinc is appropriate, and in which men the mineral may be the most beneficial.

If you believe your diet isn't giving you all of the nutrients you need, there's certainly no harm in taking a daily multivitamin and mineral supplement. However, most doctors don't recommend taking individual supplements for the sole purpose of reducing your risk of prostate disease. Not enough is known yet about the role of vitamins and minerals in preventing disease, or at what dosage they should be taken. High doses of some vitamins and minerals can be toxic.

Talk with your doctor or a registered dietitian about supplements and what best meets your needs.

## Garlic

In areas of the world where people eat a great deal of garlic, there's less prostate cancer and there's less cancer in general. One theory is that sulfur compounds in garlic enhance immune function, helping fight off disease. Sulfur may also slow the spread of cancer cells and increase the production of enzymes that help eliminate cancer-causing substances. Using fresh garlic to enhance the flavor of meats and adding it to vegetable-based sauces are easy ways to include more garlic in your diet.

## Skip the fat

Several studies suggest that there's a link between a high-calorie, high-fat diet and the development of prostate cancer. In one study, researchers at the Fred Hutchinson Cancer Research Center in Seattle found a link between a high-calorie intake and an increased risk of both localized and nonlocalized prostate cancer. They also found a link between high-fat diets and nonlocalized prostate cancer.

It's still uncertain whether the relationship between a high-fat diet and the development of cancer is due to the total amount of fat in your diet or to a specific type of fat. It's also difficult to distinguish between the effect of fat and the effect of calories. Further complicating the analysis is the fact that high-fat foods also tend to be high in calories.

Until some of these questions are answered, the basic message is, the less fat and the fewer calories you consume, the better.

## Go for the grains, fruits and vegetables

The best way to reduce fat and calories in your diet is to eat more plant-based foods. Plant foods — fruits, vegetables and foods made from whole grains — contain beneficial vitamins, minerals, fibers and cancer-protective compounds called phytochemicals. By emphasizing plant foods in your diet, you limit fat and increase the consumption of healthy compounds.

Here are the recommended types and amounts of foods to eat every day:

## Dairy products and prostate cancer

According to the American Institute for Cancer Research (AICR), a heated debate continues as to whether there is a link between milk consumption and prostate cancer. Some studies indicate that a high-calcium intake from dairy products may increase the risk of prostate cancer, but other studies dispute this.

The AICR concludes that there is insufficient evidence to prove or disprove a connection. But it says that more research is needed to help determine if the fat or calcium or some other component in dairy products may increase the risk of prostate cancer. Because of the important nutrients in dairy products, the AICR suggests that men at risk of prostate cancer make healthy choices such as low-fat or fat-free milk and yogurt a small part of a diet centered on vegetables, fruits, whole grains and beans.

**Fruits and vegetables: 8 to 10 servings.** Eating more fruits and vegetables may be one of the best things you can do to improve your overall health. In addition to being virtually fat-free and low in calories, fruits and vegetables provide fiber and a variety of nutrients, including potassium and magnesium. They also contain phytochemicals, substances that may help reduce your risk of cardiovascular disease and some cancers.

Substituting fruits and vegetables for foods that have more fat and calories is a relatively easy way to improve your diet without cutting back on the amount you eat. The key is not to smother your fruits and vegetables with dips or sauces that contain a lot of fat.

**Carbohydrates: 4 to 8 servings.** These include grains — breads, cereals, rice and pasta. Whole grains provide more fiber and nutrients, such as magnesium, than refined varieties provide. In addition to being low in fat, carbohydrates are rich in complex nutrients.

Breads and pasta are naturally low in fat and calories. To keep them that way, be selective about what you add to these foods. Avoid cream and cheese sauces on pasta and choose instead vegetable or fresh tomato-based sauces. Select plain yeast breads rather than quick breads, sweet rolls or other baked goods with added fat.

**Protein/Dairy: 4 to 7 servings.** This group contains foods from

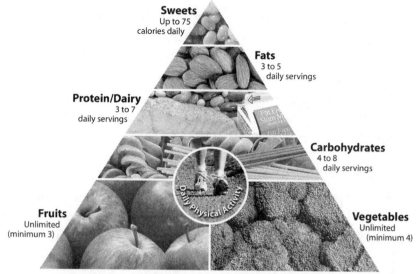

**Mayo Clinic Healthy Weight Pyramid**

both plant and animal sources. Plant-based foods rich in protein include legumes such as beans, peas and lentils. Animal-based foods rich in protein include fish and seafood, poultry, meat, eggs and dairy products such as milk and cheese. Servings are small: one serving equals 1/2 cup beans, 3 ounces fish, 1.5 to 2 ounces poultry or meat, 1 cup milk or 1.5 ounces cheese.

**Fats, sweets and alcohol: Sparingly.** Alcohol, fats and sugars provide calories but no nutrients. An obvious way to cut fat in your diet is to reduce the amount of pure fat — butter, margarine and vegetable oil — you add to food during cooking. In addition, limit sweets, such as candy, desserts and sugar-sweetened soft drinks.

## Be active

It's well known that regular exercise can help prevent a heart attack and conditions such as high blood pressure and high cholesterol. When it comes to cancer, the data isn't as clear-cut. However, studies indicate that regular exercise may reduce your cancer risk, including prostate cancer.

Exercise has been shown to strengthen your immune system, improve circulation and speed digestion — all of which may play a role in cancer prevention. Exercise also helps to prevent obesity, another potential risk factor for some cancers. Regular exercise may also reduce your risk of BPH or minimize your symptoms. Men who are physically active usually have less severe symptoms than do men who get little exercise.

If you're recovering from surgery or another treatment, be sure to talk with your doctor before beginning any physical activity program (see "Before you get started").

**Are you fit?**

More than 60 percent of American adults don't get enough physical activity to provide health benefits, and more than 25 percent aren't physically active at all during their leisure time. Federal guidelines recommend that you get either 30 to 60 minutes of moderate physical activity at least five days a week or 20 minutes of vigorous activity at least three times a week.

If you sit most of the day, you're probably not fit. Other signs that you're not as fit as you should be include:

- Feeling tired most of the time
- Being unable to keep up with others your age
- Avoiding physical activity because you tire quickly

---

## Before you get started

It's a good idea to talk with your doctor before starting a physical activity program. If you have another health problem or you're at risk of heart disease, you may need to take some special precautions while you exercise.

It's important that you see your doctor if you:

- Have blood pressure of 140/90 millimeters of mercury or higher
- Have diabetes or heart, lung or kidney disease
- Are a man age 40 years or older, or a woman age 50 years or older, and haven't had a recent physical examination
- Have a family history of heart-related problems before age 55
- Are unsure of your health status
- Have experienced chest discomfort, shortness of breath, or dizziness during exercise or strenuous activity

- Becoming short of breath or fatigued when you walk a short distance

**How to shape up**

Even if you've never exercised before in your life, it's never too late to start. You can become more fit by exercising regularly.

Three types of exercise can improve your health and, when combined with a healthy diet, possibly prevent prostate disease or reduce your symptoms. To receive the most benefit from your efforts, include a variety of activities in your exercise routine.

**Aerobic exercises.** Aerobic activities increase your breathing and heart rate and improve the health of your circulatory system, including your heart and lungs. They also build stamina and help strengthen your immune system. Try to do at least 30 minutes of aerobic activity most, if not all, days of the week. If you can't exercise for 30 minutes at a time, aim for three 10-minute sessions.

Walking is the most common aerobic activity because it's easy, convenient and inexpensive. All you need is a good pair of walking shoes. Other aerobic exercises include:

- Bicycling
- Golfing (walking, not riding)
- Volleyball
- Hiking
- Skiing
- Tennis

- Basketball
- Dancing
- Aerobic dance
- Jogging
- Running
- Swimming

## Borg Ratings of Perceived Exertion (RPE) Scale

*Perceived exertion* refers to the total amount of effort, physical stress and fatigue you experience during a physical activity. For the activity to be beneficial to your health, aim for a rating of 13 — somewhat hard. This is considered nearly ideal for most people.

| | | |
|---|---|---|
| 6 No exertion at all | 11 Light | 16 |
| 7 Extremely light | 12 | 17 Very hard |
| 8 | 13 Somewhat hard | 18 |
| 9 Very light | 14 | 19 Extremely hard |
| 10 | 15 Hard (heavy) | 20 Maximal exertion |

© 1998 Gunnar Borg

**Flexibility exercises.** Stretching before and after aerobic activity increases the range in which you can bend and stretch your joints, muscles and ligaments. Flexibility exercises also help prevent joint pain and injury. The stretches should be gentle and slow. Stretch only until you feel slight tension in your muscles. Continue to breathe normally while stretching.

Here are four stretches you can try:

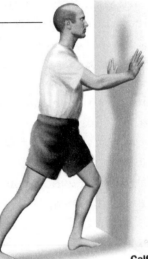

**Calf stretch**

*Calf stretch.* Stand at arm's length from the wall. Lean your upper body into the wall. Place one leg forward with knee bent. Keep your other leg back with your knee straight and your heel down. Keeping your back straight, move your hips toward the wall until you feel a stretch. Hold for 30 seconds. Relax. Repeat with the other leg.

---

## Reducing the risks of exercise

Most risks of exercise stem from doing too much, too vigorously, with too little previous conditioning. To reduce risks:

**Start out slowly.** Don't overdo it. Gradually increase your time and pace. To build up to 30 minutes, start with 10 minutes, and increase your time in five-minute increments. If you have trouble talking to a companion during your workout, you're probably pushing too hard.

**Exercise regularly and moderately.** Never exercise to the point of nausea, dizziness, severe shortness of breath, heart palpitations, or tightness or pain in your chest. If you experience any of these symptoms, stop exercising and get immediate medical care.

**Always warm up and cool down.** This reduces stress on your heart and muscles.

*Upper-thigh stretch.* Lie on your back on a table or bed, with one leg and hip as near the edge as possible. Let your lower leg hang relaxed over the edge. Grasp the knee of your other leg, and pull your thigh and knee firmly toward your chest until

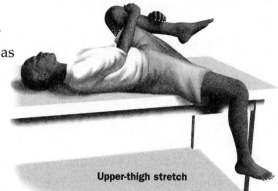

**Upper-thigh stretch**

your lower back flattens against the table or bed. Hold for 30 seconds. Relax. Repeat with the other leg.

*Chest stretch.* Clasp your hands behind your head. Pull your elbows firmly back while inhaling deeply. Hold for 30 seconds. Relax.

**Chest stretch**

*Low back stretch.* Lie flat on a firm surface. With your knees bent, lift one leg at a time toward your body. Grasp your knees and pull toward your shoulders. Stop when you feel a stretch in your lower back. Hold. Return legs, one at a time, to starting position. Repeat. Avoid this exercise if you have osteoporosis or an artificial hip implant.

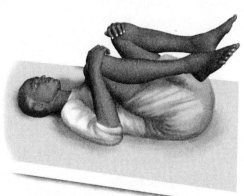

**Low back stretch**

**Strengthening exercises.** They build stronger muscles to improve posture, balance and coordination. They also promote healthy bones and increase your metabolism, which can help keep your weight in check. Add strengthening exercises to your routine at least twice a week. Start with five repetitions of each and try to build up to 25 repetitions.

Here are six strengthening exercises you can try:

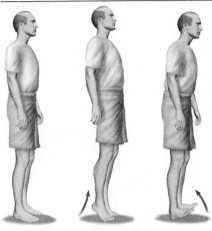

*Toe and heel raise.* Standing, rise up so that your weight is on your toes. Then rock back and shift your weight to your heels, lifting your toes off the ground. This strengthens your calf and lower leg muscles to improve your balance.

**Toe and heel raise**

*Abdominal exercise No. 1.* Lie on a firm surface with your knees bent. Flatten the small of your back against the surface and concentrate on tightening your abdominal muscles. Relax and repeat.

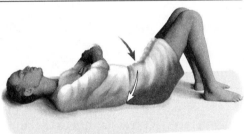

**Abdominal exercise No. 1**

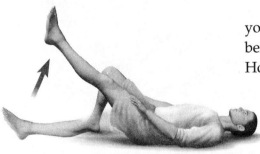

**Abdominal exercise No. 2**

*Abdominal exercise No. 2.* Lie on your back with your right knee bent and your left knee straight. Hold your abdominal muscles tight, and slowly raise and lower your left leg. Relax and repeat. Reverse legs. Avoid doing abdominal exercise if you have osteoporosis.

*Wall push-ups.* Face the wall and stand far enough away so that you can place your palms on the wall and your elbows are slightly bent. Slowly bend your elbows and lean toward the wall, supporting your weight with your arms. Straighten your arms and return to your starting position. As you build strength, try standing farther away from the wall.

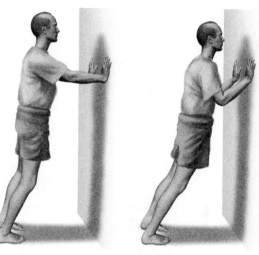

**Wall push-ups**

*Wall slide.* Stand with your heels about 12 inches (30.5 centimeters) from the wall. With your back against the wall, slowly slide down the surface until your knees are bent at a 45-degree angle. Slide back up to a standing position. This strengthens your quadriceps, improving walking and climbing strength.

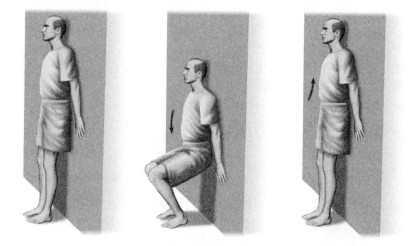

**Wall slide**

*Arm curl.* Stand with your feet shoulder-width apart. For resistance, hold a partially filled half-gallon milk jug. Flex your elbow until your hand reaches shoulder height. Hold, then lower your arm slowly. This tones your biceps and helps in carrying and lifting. Remember to keep your wrist rigid while lifting — don't bend or curl your wrist.

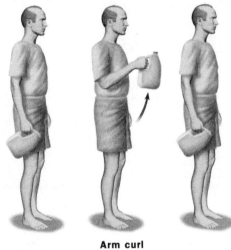

**Arm curl**

### Keeping your program on track

The following tips can help you stay physically active and keep up your motivation:

**Set goals.** Start with simple goals and then progress to longer-range goals. People who can stay physically active for six months usually end up making regular activity a habit. Make your goals realistic and achievable. It's easy to get frustrated and give up on goals that are too ambitious.

**Add variety.** Vary what you do to prevent boredom. For example, try alternating walking and bicycling with swimming or a low-impact aerobics class. On days when the weather is pleasant, do your flexibility or strengthening exercises outside. Consider joining a health club to access different forms of physical activity.

**Track your progress.** Record what you do each time you exercise, how long you do it, and how you feel during and after exercising. Recording your efforts helps you work toward your goals and reminds you that you're making progress.

**Reward yourself.** Work on developing an internal reward that comes from feelings of accomplishment, self-esteem and control of your own behavior. After each activity session, take two to five minutes to sit down and relax. Savor the good feelings that exercise gives you and think about what you've just accomplished. This type of internal reward can help you make a long-term commitment to regular exercise.

## See your doctor regularly

An annual prostate checkup can't reduce your risk of cancer, BPH or prostatitis, as perhaps a healthy diet or exercise can. But having regular checkups is crucial to staying healthy. If prostate disease does develop, a digital rectal exam or prostate-specific antigen (PSA) test often can catch the problem in its earliest stages, when it's the easiest to treat and cure. If you don't regularly see a doctor, schedule an appointment to have a physical examination, including a prostate exam, and make it a yearly habit.

If you experience prostate-related signs and symptoms — increased urination, difficulty urinating, pain while urinating, lower pelvic and back pain, or blood in your urine or semen — have them attended to as soon as possible, even if you think that it's nothing. You don't want to risk the possibility that you could be wrong.

## Answers to your questions

*Does alcohol play a role in the risk of prostate disease?*
There's no evidence that a moderate amount of alcohol causes prostate disease. A moderate amount of alcohol for men is two drinks a day, one drink a day if you're 65 or older. However, if you regularly drink more than a moderate amount of alcohol, this may interfere with your diet. People who drink excessive amounts of alcohol often substitute alcohol for food and may not get adequate amounts of nutrients. A poor diet can weaken your immune system and reduce your body's natural defenses against disease.

*Is soy sauce a good source of soy?*
No. Soy sauce doesn't contain beneficial amounts of cancer-fighting chemicals, and it's very high in sodium. If you're sensitive to sodium, regular use of soy sauce can increase your blood pressure.

*Is it true that stress can cause prostate problems?*
It hasn't been proved that stress increases your risk of prostate disease, but there's some evidence that stress may play a role. Stress weakens your immune system, making it more difficult for your body to fight off disease, including cancer. Researchers also theorize that stress can produce tension in your lower pelvic muscles, affecting normal functioning of the prostate gland and, possibly, causing prostatitis.

## Chapter 12

# What about complementary and alternative therapies?

As Americans take a more active role in their health care, many are exploring options for their care that fall outside the realm of traditional medicine. You may be among this growing group. Perhaps you've purchased an herbal supplement at your local health food store. Or you may have tried yoga, meditation or acupuncture.

Complementary and alternative medicine covers a broad range of healing philosophies, approaches and therapies. Although the two terms are often used synonymously, they aren't the same.

The National Center for Complementary and Alternative Medicine (NCCAM), a division of the National Institutes of Health, defines complementary medicine as unconventional medical practices used *in addition to* those treatments recommended by your doctor. An example is using tai chi in addition to prescription medicine to manage anxiety. NCCAM defines alternative medicine as treatments used *in place of* traditional medicine. This might include seeing a homeopathic or naturopathic practitioner for your health care.

The question is, do these therapies work? Some do show promise and are slowly gaining acceptance within mainstream medicine. But the benefits of many products and practices remain unproved.

Here's a look at some of the more common complementary and alternative treatments promoted for prevention or treatment of prostate disease, and cancer in general.

## Dietary and herbal supplements

As anyone who has walked through a health food store can attest, the profusion of dietary supplements and herbal remedies is almost overwhelming. Literally thousands of products crowd the shelves, touting all sorts of claims.

Herbal products marketed to relieve common prostate problems, such as frequent urination or a weak urine flow, include:

- Pygeum (*Pygeum africanum*): also known as African plum tree
- African wild potato (*Hypoxis rooperi*): also known as South African star grass
- Pumpkin (*Cucurbita pepo*) seeds
- Rye grass (*Secale cereale*)
- Stinging nettle — above ground parts (*Urtica dioica* and *Urtica urens*): also known as common nettle

Taken in small to moderate amounts, these products appear safe. However, they haven't been studied in large, long-term trials to confirm their safety or to prove they work.

An exception is the herb saw palmetto (*Serenoa repens*). Unlike other herbal supplements, it has been widely tested, and the results show promise.

### Saw palmetto

Saw palmetto is made from the berries of the saw palmetto plant, found in southern Florida. Hundreds of years ago, Seminoles used the plant as an aphrodisiac. In recent decades, it has become a popular treatment for reducing the symptoms of benign prostatic hyperplasia (BPH). In Europe, saw palmetto is sold as a drug. In the United States, it's available as an herbal supplement in health food stores.

Saw palmetto is thought to work by preventing testosterone from being converted into a form of the hormone associated with prostate tissue growth. In 1998, researchers with the Department of Veterans Affairs reviewed more than a dozen studies involving saw palmetto,

## Using saw palmetto

Future studies may provide more information about the best use of this herbal supplement. In the meantime, the *Natural Medicines Comprehensive Database* offers the following guidelines if you choose to take saw palmetto:

**Effectiveness.** Saw palmetto is likely to be effective when used orally for reducing the symptoms of benign prostatic hyperplasia (BPH). However, it doesn't reduce prostate enlargement.

**Adverse reactions.** The adverse reactions of saw palmetto are generally mild. Dizziness, gastrointestinal problems such as nausea, vomiting, constipation and diarrhea are the most frequently reported side effects. Saw palmetto may increase clotting time and caution is advised when taking it with anti-coagulant or antiplatelet medications.

Adapted from: *Natural Medicines Comprehensive Database*, 2003

and concluded that the herb appears to be as effective as the medication finasteride (Proscar), and with fewer side effects. However, the researchers recommended additional studies to determine the appropriate daily dose of the supplement and its long-term effectiveness. Other studies have produced similar results.

Saw palmetto works slowly. Most men begin to see an improvement in their urinary symptoms within one to three months. If after three months you haven't noticed any benefit from the product, then it may not work for you.

It appears safe to take saw palmetto indefinitely, but possible side effects from long-term use are unknown. It had been thought that taking saw palmetto could suppress prostate-specific antigen (PSA) levels in your blood, rendering results of a PSA test inaccurate. But recent studies have shown that taking saw palmetto has no effect on PSA levels.

### Cancer-fighting supplements

A few herbal and dietary products claim to help cure or prevent cancer. There's no scientific evidence that these products work, and some may be dangerous. Three popular supplements that are sold as cancer-fighting agents are:

**Chaparral.** Also known as creosote bush or greasewood, chaparral (*Larrea tridentata*) comes from a desert shrub found in the southwestern United States and Mexico. American Indians first used chaparral to treat ailments from the common cold to snakebites. In recent decades, the herb has been formulated into teas, capsules and tablets, with claims it can cure a number of disorders and diseases, including cancer.

Researchers believe a chemical in chaparral called nordihydroguaiaretic acid may prevent replication of cancer cells, as well as viruses and bacteria. However, studies of chaparral haven't shown that the herb destroys or prevents cancer, and research suggests it can lead to irreversible liver failure.

**PC-SPES.** This was an herbal mixture marketed for treatment of prostate cancer containing eight herbs — *Dendranthema morifolium, Ganoderma lucidum, Glycyrrhiza glabra* (licorice), *Isatis indigotica, Panax pseudoginseng, Rabdosia rubescens, Scutellaria baicalensis* and *Seronoa repens* (saw palmetto). A study of PC-SPES published in the *New England Journal of Medicine* in 1998 found that the product worked like estrogen supplements. It reduced concentrations of testosterone that promoted prostate cancer growth, and in some instances may have suppressed the cancer, at least temporarily. However, the product commonly produced impotence and breast tenderness. It also caused blood clots in deep leg veins and, if taken in large amounts, could be toxic.

However, this and other PC-SPES studies became suspect when laboratory analysis found that several batches of PC-SPES were contaminated with pharmaceutical drugs, including an estrogen preparation and the blood thinner warfarin. The manufacturer voluntarily pulled the product from the market in 2002, and the Food and Drug Administration (FDA) issued a warning to consumers to stop taking it. Whether the promising results obtained early on with PC-SPES were due to the herbs or simply the result of added estrogen is unclear. For now, PC-SPES remains off the market.

**Shark cartilage.** Some researchers believe that shark cartilage contains a protein that inhibits the formation of new blood vessels

# Cancer help or hype?

Supplements are just one form of unconventional treatment for cancer. Other practices include:

**Chelation therapy.** A doctor injects a chelating agent into your bloodstream. The agent is thought to bind to certain elements like lead, mercury and other potentially cancer-causing substances, eliminating them from your bloodstream. Another theory is that chelation improves overall circulation, increasing the amount of oxygen delivered to your cells. Cancer is thought to grow better in the absence of oxygen.

Chelation is an approved treatment for people with heavy-metal toxicity, but no evidence shows that it can treat other diseases, including cancer. The therapy can also produce significant side effects, including kidney and bone marrow damage, an irregular heart rhythm, and severe inflammation of the veins. It should only be performed by a knowledgeable doctor.

**Macrobiotics.** This healing therapy requires that you follow a specific diet, in addition to certain lifestyle practices. The diet consists of whole grains, vegetables, sea vegetables, beans and soybean-based soups. Lifestyle practices include maintaining a positive mental outlook and strong personal relationships, getting plenty of exercise, wearing natural fabrics, and cooking with utensils made from natural products, such as wood, glass and ceramic.

The philosophy behind macrobiotics is that natural foods, utensils and fabrics, combined with a positive attitude and social interconnectedness, promote health and harmony and fight disease, including cancer. However, there's no evidence macrobiotics prevents or cures cancer. The diet itself has many health benefits, including being low in fat and high in certain vitamins, minerals and phytochemcials. It is deficient in other nutrients, though, and may require supplemental nutrients to balance its shortcomings.

within tumors, preventing cancer in sharks. Shark cartilage therapy is based on the theory that capsules containing shark cartilage will do the same in humans — stop and shrink cancerous tumors. But in limited studies, shark cartilage supplements have generally been found to be ineffective.

Among other things, it's doubtful that the capsules contain enough purified protein to have any effect. Also, your stomach and intestines may digest the protein, just as they do other proteins, so it may never get to your bloodstream to be of help. In addition to tasting bad, high doses of shark cartilage can produce nausea in some people.

### Knowing the risks

Unlike the medications your doctor prescribes, the FDA doesn't regulate the effectiveness of dietary and herbal products. In addition, regulations regarding the safety of these products differ from those of the FDA. With prescription drugs, the manufacturer must prove that the benefits of the drug outweigh any safety concerns before the drug is approved for sale. However, with dietary and herbal supplements, health officials assume the products are safe until they're proven otherwise. Only when a supplement is shown to be unsafe is it removed from the market. Because these products are not subject to the same safety procedures as prescription drugs, they can contain toxic substances that may not be listed on the label. Their dosages also can vary.

In addition, just because a product is "natural" doesn't mean it's safe. Poisonous mushrooms, for example, are natural. But when eaten, they can cause serious illness and even death.

Because it's not always easy to tell which products may be unsafe or a waste of your money, the best advice is to talk with your doctor before taking any dietary or herbal product.

## Mind and body therapies

These practices are based on the interrelationship of the mind and body, and the power of one to affect the other. Mind and body therapies are most commonly used to relieve anxiety and stress and to promote an overall sense of well-being. Some evidence shows that they may also strengthen your immune system. Mind and body therapies can't cure prostate disease, but some people find the therapies helpful in coping with the emotional and physical effects of cancer.

## Humor therapy

Humor therapy is based on the belief that frequent periods of laughter help distract your attention from health problems. Laughter is also a kind of analgesic. It promotes the release of chemicals that fight pain, as well as reduce depression.

Humor therapy simply involves lightening your day with some laughter. You might watch a funny movie, call a friend who makes you laugh, joke with your neighbors or co-workers, or visit a comedy club.

## Hypnosis

People have been using hypnosis to promote healing since ancient times. In the past 50 years, there has been a resurgence of interest in hypnosis among some physicians, psychologists and mental health professionals.

Hypnosis produces an induced state of relaxation in which your mind stays focused and open to suggestion. No one knows how hypnosis works, but experts believe it alters brain wave patterns in much the same way as other relaxation techniques.

During a therapy session, you receive suggestions designed to help you decrease stress and anxiety and increase your ability to cope with your medical condition. Unlike situations sometimes portrayed in movies and on television, you can't be forced under hypnosis to do something you normally wouldn't want to do. Approximately 75 percent of adults can be hypnotized by a trained professional. People who don't want to feel out of control often can't be hypnotized.

## Meditation

Meditation is a way to calm your mind and body, originating in religious and cultural traditions. During meditation you sit quietly and focus on nothing or on a mantra — a simple sound repeated over and over. This causes you to enter a deeply restful state which reduces your body's stress response. Your breathing slows, your muscles relax, and your brain wave activity indicates a state of relaxation.

Regular meditation can help reduce anxiety and stress. Studies suggest it may also reduce blood pressure and possibly even promote longevity.

Although meditation may sound simple, learning to control your thoughts isn't easy. The more you practice, though, the easier it gets to concentrate without having your mind wander.

### Music, dance and art therapy

These therapies include graceful dancing, art expression and performing or listening to music. In addition to their calming and soothing effects, they can help promote self-confidence and personal well-being, and may reduce symptoms of depression.

Several national organizations promote the use of music, dance and art for health and healing, with chapters set up across the country. Some medical centers also offer music, dance or art therapy programs.

### Yoga

Yoga is a 5,000-year-old practice that incorporates proper breathing, movement and posture to achieve a union of mind, body and spirit. It involves completing a series of positions, during which you pay special attention to your breathing — exhaling during certain movements and inhaling with others.

Yoga may help control stress, anxiety and pain. However, to be effective, yoga requires training and regular practice.

## Traditional Chinese medicine

Some complementary and alternative therapies center on the belief that natural energy forces play an important role in overall health and healing. Many of these therapies are based on ancient Chinese philosophies. There's no proof that these therapies can treat prostate disease, but they do appear to be safe, and they may provide other health benefits.

## Acupressure

Acupressure, like acupuncture, stems from the Chinese belief that just below your skin are 14 invisible pathways, called meridians. Through these pathways flows *chi*, or *qi* (chee), the Chinese term for "the body's life force." When the flow of chi is interrupted, illness results.

During acupressure, a practitioner applies pressure with his or her finger to specific points on your body to restore the free flow of chi and relieve your symptoms. Research on the benefits of acupressure is inconclusive. Many people who feel they're helped by the procedure find its hands-on therapy to be relaxing.

## Acupuncture

Acupuncture is one of the most studied nontraditional medical practices, and it's gaining acceptance in Western medicine for the treatment of certain conditions. A consensus statement on acupuncture released in 1998 by the National Institutes of Health states there's enough evidence to prove that acupuncture helps relieve dental pain after surgery, and nausea caused by chemotherapy, anesthesia or pregnancy. For other conditions, evidence of the procedure's benefits is less clear. However, several studies indicate that acupuncture may be effective for the relief of cancer pain.

During a typical acupuncture session, an acupuncturist inserts one to 10 hair-thin needles into your skin for 15 to 40 minutes. The purpose of the needles is to remove blockages and promote the free flow of chi. The acupuncturist may also manipulate the needles or apply electrical stimulation or heat to the needles. Insertion of the needles should cause little or no pain. Some people even find the procedure relaxing.

Adverse side effects from acupuncture are rare, but they can occur. Make sure your acupuncturist is trained and follows good hygienic practices, including the use of disposable needles.

## Tai chi

Tai chi (TIE-chee) is a series of self-defense postures and exercises developed in China more than 1,000 years ago. No longer used to ward off enemies, tai chi has become an increasingly popular practice — especially among older adults — for strengthening muscles, improving flexibility and reducing stress.

Tai chi involves gentle, deliberate circular movements, combined with deep breathing. As you concentrate on the motions of your body, you develop a feeling of tranquility. "Moving meditation" is how people who practice tai chi sometimes describe it. Similar to other forms of Chinese medicine, it's designed to foster the free flow of chi necessary for health.

## Other approaches to healing

These practices attempt to cure and prevent illness through different — and controversial — routes. Studies are limited on the effectiveness of these approaches, and their benefits generally remain unproved:

### Ayurveda
This healing philosophy stems from medical practices in India, and is becoming more popular in the United States. Ayurveda (AH-yer-vay-duh) is based on the principle that mind and body are one and that the body cannot be well if the mind is troubled.

Ayurveda practitioners believe that cancer stems from emotional, spiritual and physical imbalances in life. To treat the cancer, you need to purge your body of toxic substances through bloodletting, vomiting or bowel emptying. You use diet, herbs, breathing exercises and massage to rebuild and maintain proper balance. There's no evidence that this practice can cure disease.

### Homeopathy
Homeopathic medicine uses highly diluted preparations of natural substances, typically plants and minerals, to treat symptoms of illness. Homeopathy is based on a "law of similars." Practitioners believe that if a large dose of a substance causes you to have certain symptoms when you're healthy, a small dose of the same substance can treat illnesses that produce the same symptoms.

Working from a list of nearly 2,000 substances, a homeopath selects the most appropriate remedy for your particular set of symptoms. Generally, you take only one preparation at a time, until you find one that relieves your symptoms.

Chronic and occasional conditions, such as arthritis, asthma, allergies, colds and influenza, are the main reasons people use homeopathic medicine. However, some homeopaths believe their remedies can cure all illnesses.

Scientific research hasn't been able to explain how or whether homeopathic medicines work. And because most homeopathic medicines are so diluted, many scientists are skeptical of their effectiveness.

### Naturopathic medicine

This form of medicine integrates traditional natural therapies, including acupuncture, manipulative therapy, herbal medicines, and nutritional therapies, with modern diagnostic sciences and standards of care. Instead of traditional medications or surgery to treat illness, naturopathic doctors rely on methods aimed at strengthening the body's natural healing ability.

To become certified, naturopathic physicians go through four years of medical training. Their training, however, is substantially different from that of traditional medical doctors.

Naturopathic physicians claim they can treat the same range of conditions as other doctors. However, these claims haven't been scientifically proved.

## How to evaluate nontraditional therapies

If you're considering using a complementary or alternative therapy, practice or product — or you already do — the National Center for Complementary and Alternative Medicine recommends that you follow these steps:

**Research the safety and effectiveness of the product or therapy.** The benefits you receive from the treatment should outweigh its risks. To find out more about a product or therapy, you can request information from the NCCAM, or visit its Web site (see "Additional resources" on page 173). You can also search the scientific literature on the product or therapy at a public or university library, or via the Internet. But be aware that many Web sites that tout health information are merely advertising fronts for various products.

**Determine the reliability of the practitioner or salesperson.** If you're working with a licensed practitioner, check with your

---

## Too good to be true?

The Food and Drug Administration and the National Council Against Health Fraud recommend that you watch for use of the following claims or practices. These are often warning signs of potentially fraudulent products or therapies:

- The advertisements or promotional materials include words such as *breakthrough, magical* or *new discovery*. If the product or therapy were in fact a cure, it would be widely reported in the media and your doctor would recommend its use.
- The product materials include pseudo medical jargon such as *detoxify, purify* or *energize*. Such descriptions are difficult to define and to measure.
- The manufacturer claims the product can treat a wide range of symptoms, or cure or prevent a number of diseases. No one product can do this.
- The product seems to be backed by scientific studies, but references for these research studies are not provided, are very limited, or are out of date. Manufacturers of legitimate products like to promote the results of scientific studies, not hide them.
- The product has no negative side effects, only benefits. Most medications and other therapies have some side effects.
- The manufacturer of the product accuses the government, medical profession or drug companies of suppressing important information about the helpfulness of the product. There's no reason for the government or medical profession to do so.

local and state medical boards for information about the person's credentials and whether any complaints have been filed against that person. If you're buying a product from a business or its representative, check with your local or state business bureau to find out whether any complaints have been filed against the company.

**Estimate the total cost of the treatment.** Because many complementary and alternative approaches aren't covered by health insurance, it's important that you know exactly how much the treatment will cost you.

**Talk with your doctor.** Your doctor can help you determine whether the treatment may be beneficial and if it's safe. Some complementary and alternative products or therapies may interfere with medications you're taking or adversely affect other health conditions you have.

**Don't substitute a proven treatment for an unproven one.** If it has been proved that medication, surgery or other treatment recommended by your doctor can help your condition, don't replace this treatment with alternative products, practices or therapies that haven't been proven effective.

## The choice is yours

Good health doesn't just happen. It generally stems from making wise choices, such as avoiding smoking, limiting alcohol use, controlling stress, and practicing safe sexual habits. Prostate health is no different.

The choices you make day in and day out can keep your prostate healthy — or help it to become healthy again. Lifestyle changes, including eating a more nutritious diet and increasing your level of physical activity, may prevent prostate disease or slow its progression. Regularly seeing your doctor and having a yearly prostate examination increase your chance of identifying prostate problems early, when they can be treated and cured. Discussing complementary and alternative therapies with your doctor reduces your risk of potentially dangerous side effects from questionable products or practices.

The fact that you're reading this book is an important first step, and an indication that you want to make the right decisions for treating or preventing prostate disease. The information and suggestions in this book can help you achieve and maintain prostate health, and live a longer, healthier life.

# Additional resources

Contact these organizations for more information about prostate conditions. Some groups offer free printed material or videotapes. Others have materials or videos that you can purchase.

### American Cancer Society

1599 Clifton Road N.E.
Atlanta, GA  30329-4250
(800) ACS-2345, or (800) 227-2345
*www.cancer.org*

### American Foundation for Urologic Disease

1128 N. Charles St.
Baltimore, MD  21201-5559
(410) 468-1800
*www.afud.org*

### American Institute for Cancer Research

1759 R St. N.W.
Washington, DC  20009
(800) 843-8114
*www.aicr.org*

### American Prostate Society

P.O Box 870
Hanover, MD  21076
(800) 308-1106
(410) 859-3735
*www.ameripros.org*

## American Urological Association

1120 Charles St.
Baltimore, MD 21201
(410) 727-1100
*www.auanet.org*

## Cancer Care

275 Seventh Ave.
New York, NY 10001
(800) 813-HOPE, or (800) 813-4673
*www.cancercare.org*

## Cancer Research Institute

681 Fifth Ave.
New York, NY 10022
(800) 992-2623
*www.cancerresearch.org*

## Centers for Disease Control and Prevention

1600 Clifton Road
Atlanta, GA 30333
(800) 311-3435
*www.cdc.gov*

## MayoClinic.com

Mayo Clinic Health Information
200 1st St. S.W.
Rochester, MN 55905
*www.MayoClinic.com*

## National Association for Continence

P.O. Box 1019
Charleston, SC 29402-1019
(800) BLADDER, or (800) 252-3337
*www.nafc.org*

## National Cancer Institute

Public Inquiries Office
6116 Executive Blvd., MSC 8322
Suite 3036A
Bethesda, MD 20892-8322
(800) 4-CANCER, or (800) 422-6237
*www.nci.nih.gov*

## National Center for Complementary and Alternative Medicine

NCCAM Clearinghouse
P.O. Box 7923
Gaithersburg, MD 20898
(888) 644-6226
*www.nccam.nih.gov*

## National Hospice and Palliative Organization

1700 Diagonal Rd.
Suite 625
Alexandria, VA 22314
(800) 646-6460
*www.nhpco.org*

## National Kidney and Urologic Disease Information Clearinghouse

3 Information Way
Bethesda, MD 20892-3580
(301) 654-4415
(800) 891-5390
*www.niddk.nih.gov/health/kidney/nkudic.htm*

## Sexual Function Health Council

American Foundation for Urologic Disease
1128 N. Charles St.
Baltimore, MD 21201-5559
(410) 468-1800
*www.afud.org*

## Us Too International

5003 Fairview Ave.
Suite 50
Downers Grove, IL 60515
(800) 80-US TOO, or (800) 808-7866
*www.ustoo.com*

# Glossary

**androgens.** Hormones, including testosterone, that are responsible for the normal development of male sex organs and other features, such as facial hair and muscles.

**antiandrogen therapy.** Medications that prevent testosterone produced in the adrenal glands from reaching prostate cancer cells.

**benign prostatic hyperplasia (BPH).** A noncancerous condition that results when tissues in the prostate gland enlarge and press on the urethra, restricting normal urine flow.

**biopsy.** A procedure in which a doctor removes a sample of tissue from your body. This sample is then examined under a microscope for signs of disease, such as cancer.

**bone scan.** A procedure in which a harmless, low-grade radioactive solution is injected into your bloodstream. The solution attaches to areas of new bone growth that may stem from cancer.

**brachytherapy.** A treatment that involves implanting radioactive seeds directly inside the prostate gland or nearby. Also known as interstitial implantation or internal radiotherapy.

**bulking agents.** Substances injected into the urethra that puff up urethral tissue and narrow the opening of your bladder. Bulking agents are used to treat incontinence.

**catheter.** A flexible, thin tube that's inserted in the body to inject or drain fluid. A catheter inserted into the penis and up the urethra allows urine to drain.

**clinical staging.** Exams and tests that are done to discover the extent of cancer within the body — both at its original site and in other parts of the body. Also called staging.

**computerized tomography (CT) scan.** Images of internal organs that are stacked together by a computer connected to an X-ray machine. The images are displayed on a screen and give a three-dimensional view of those organs from any angle.

**cryotherapy.** A procedure in which a doctor injects extremely cold liquid nitrogen into an organ, such as the prostate. The nitrogen freezes and kills abnormal cells.

**cystitis.** Inflammation of the bladder, often due to infection. Cystitis can lead to painful urination.

**digital rectal examination (DRE).** A procedure in which a doctor inserts a gloved finger into your rectum to examine the prostate. A prostate that feels abnormal may have some form of disease.

**ejaculation.** The release of semen through the penis that occurs during male orgasm.

**estrogen.** A hormone produced primarily in females that helps the body to produce feminine physical characteristics, menstruation and changes related to pregnancy. As a medication for prostate cancer, estrogen is used to block the activity of testosterone.

**external beam therapy.** Radiation therapy delivered with a machine that produces high-energy rays, such as X-rays, to kill cancer cells. Also called external radiotherapy, in contrast with internal radiotherapy.

**Gleason grading system.** A way to describe the extent of prostate cancer, named for the system's creator, Donald Gleason, M.D. The system is a scale that goes from 1 to 5, with 1 being the least aggressive form of cancer.

**gynecomastia.** Excessive growth of male breasts due to lack of testosterone. This is sometimes a side effect of hormone deprivation therapy.

**heat therapy (thermotherapy).** Treatment that uses computer-controlled heat to destroy excessive prostate tissue.

**hematospermia.** The presence of blood in the semen.

**hematuria.** The presence of blood in the urine.

**hormone.** A substance secreted by an endocrine gland and carried through the bloodstream. Hormones regulate many body functions and can play a role in the development of cancer.

**hormone deprivation therapy.** Treatment with drugs or surgery that reduces the supply of male sex hormones and prevents them from reaching a cancer. Also called androgen deprivation therapy.

**impotence.** A man's inability to achieve or keep an erection and engage in sexual intercourse.

**incontinence (urinary).** Inability to control the release of urine.

**indolent.** Describes type of disease, such as prostate cancer, that grows slowly and produces few symptoms.

**interstitial laser therapy.** A treatment for benign prostatic hyperplasia (BPH) that directs laser energy to the inside of a benign tumor. The aim is to reduce the volume of the prostate and increase urinary flow.

**Kegel exercises.** Voluntary movement of your pelvic floor muscles to improve their condition and tone. Kegel exercises can help to reduce mild to moderate incontinence.

**laparoscopy.** Surgery done to examine the inside of your abdomen with a laparoscope and remove lymph nodes suspected of containing cancer from your pelvic area. A laparoscope is a thin, lighted tube that contains a tiny fiber-optic camera.

**latent.** Describes a condition that is present in your body but inactive, producing no symptoms.

**LH-RH agonist.** A medication that interrupts the activity of LH-RH. As a result, your testicles never get the message to produce testosterone.

**luteinizing-hormone-releasing hormone (LH-RH).** A hormone that alerts the pituitary gland to release luteinizing hormone (LH). In turn, LH signals your testicles to make testosterone.

**lymph node biopsy.** Surgery to remove lymph nodes so that they can be examined for signs of cancer.

**lymph nodes.** Small, bean-shaped structures throughout your body that produce white blood cells. These cells help to protect you from harmful bacteria and other organisms.

**magnetic resonance imaging (MRI).** A procedure that uses strong magnetic fields to produce detailed images of areas inside your body.

**maximum androgen blockade.** Treatment designed to stop your body from producing male hormones. This treatment can include hormone medications or surgery to remove the testicles.

**metastatic prostate cancer.** Abnormal cell growth that has spread from the prostate to lymph nodes or other areas of your body.

**needle biopsy.** A procedure in which a surgeon inserts a small needle into an organ, such as the prostate gland. Using the needle, the surgeon removes a sample of your tissue, which is examined in a laboratory for signs of cancer.

**orchiectomy.** Surgery to remove the testicles, which prevents the production of testosterone. Hormone-blocking drugs have reduced the need for testicular surgery. Also called castration.

**palpable tumor.** An abnormal growth of tissue that can be felt, or palpated.

**pelvic lymph node dissection.** A procedure in which a surgeon removes lymph nodes located near the prostate. A pathologist examines the lymph nodes to discover whether prostate cancer has spread.

**perineal prostatectomy.** A procedure in which a surgeon makes an incision in the perineum to remove the prostate gland.

**perineum.** In a man, the space between the scrotum and the anus.

**proctitis.** An inflamed rectum, often occurring with bleeding, diarrhea and pain.

**prostate gland.** An organ that is located just below a man's bladder and surrounds the top of the urethra. This gland produces most of the fluids in semen.

**prostatic intraepithelial neoplasia (PIN).** Abnormal prostate cells that may signal the presence of cancer, or the increased chance that cancer will be found on a later biopsy. PIN is usually divided into low and high grade indicating the degree of risk.

**prostate-specific antigen (PSA).** A protein produced by the prostate gland that can be measured in the blood. A PSA test can determine how much of this protein is circulating in your blood. PSA comes in two forms — that which is bound to blood proteins, and that which is unbound, called free PSA. Conditions other than cancer can increase your PSA levels.

**prostatic stent.** A tiny metal coil that is inserted into the urethra to widen the urethra and keep it open.

**prostatitis.** A general term for inflammation of the prostate gland.

**radiation oncologist.** A specialist in cancer treatment who performs radiation therapy.

**radiation therapy.** The use of radiation — either with an external beam or internal implants — to kill cancer cells.

**radical prostatectomy.** A procedure in which a surgeon removes your entire prostate gland, usually along with some nearby tissue. Retropubic surgery involves an incision in the lower abdomen. Perineal surgery uses an incision between the anus and the scrotal sac.

**semen.** A thick, whitish fluid containing sperm cells. Men discharge this fluid from the penis during orgasm.

**seminal vesicles.** Sac-like glands located behind the bladder in men. These structures secrete fluid that becomes part of semen.

**sperm.** Male reproductive cells that are produced in the testicles and transmitted in semen.

**staging.** See clinical staging.

**surgical margins.** The borders of tissue that's cut and removed during surgery. One goal of prostate cancer surgery is to remove the prostate gland in a way that leaves behind tissue edges (margins) free of cancer.

**testicles.** The egg-shaped glands in the scrotum that produce sperm as well as testosterone.

**testosterone.** A male sex hormone produced in the testicles. Testosterone is an androgen that can promote the growth of prostate cancer.

**three-dimensional conformal radiation therapy (3D-CRT).** Radiation therapy that uses computer software to produce three-dimensional images of an organ, such as the prostate gland. These images allow a therapist to direct radiation beams so that they correspond to the shape of the organ — sparing normal tissue located nearby.

**TNM rating system.** A method for describing the extent of a cancer. T stands for tumor and signifies the extent of the cancer in, and adjacent to, the prostate gland. N stands for nodes and signifies whether the cancer has spread to nearby lymph nodes. M stands for metastasis — cancer that has spread to other tissues or organs.

**transrectal ultrasound (TRUS).** The use of sound waves that are bounced off the prostate and converted by a computer into an image of the prostate.

**transurethral electrovaporization of the prostate (TUVP).** A form of heat therapy involving a metal instrument that emits a high-frequency electrical current. A doctor uses this instrument to remove excess tissue from the prostate.

**transurethral incision of the prostate (TUIP).** A procedure in which a surgeon makes one or two small cuts in the prostate gland. The cuts enlarge the opening of the urethra, making it easier to urinate.

**transurethral microwave therapy (TUMT).** A form of heat therapy that uses computer-controlled microwave energy to destroy the inner portion of an enlarged prostate gland.

**transurethral needle ablation (TUNA).** A form of heat therapy that works by sending radio waves through needles that are inserted into the prostate gland. These waves destroy excess tissue.

**transurethral resection of the prostate (TURP).** A procedure in which a surgeon threads a narrow instrument into the urethra and uses small cutting tools to scrape away excess prostate tissue.

**tumor.** An abnormal growth of tissue. The growth may be cancerous (malignant) or not cancerous (benign).

**tumor markers.** Substances circulating in the blood that are produced by tumors. The level of a tumor marker may reflect the extent of the tumor.

**ureters.** The tubes that carry urine from your kidneys to your bladder.

**urethra.** The tube extending from the bladder to the tip of the penis. The urethra carries urine from the bladder. During ejaculation, the urethra transports semen from the prostate gland.

**urologist.** A doctor who specializes in treating disorders of the urinary and reproductive systems in men.

**vasa deferentia.** Two tubes that carry sperm from the testicles to the prostate gland and urethra. These are severed during a prostatectomy.

**visual laser ablation of the prostate (VLAP).** A treatment that applies laser energy to dry up and destroy excess cells in the prostate gland.

**watchful waiting.** The decision to hold off on aggressive treatment and observe your condition to see if it changes.

# Index

*Note:* Glossary definitions are indicated by the **boldface** page numbers.

# "No. 1 book of its kind"
— *U.S. News & World Report*

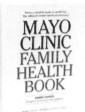

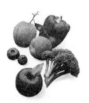

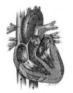

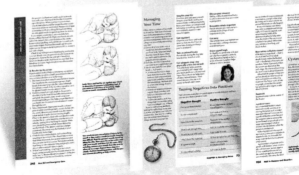
*A question of health? Mayo Clinic books are the answer.*